STUDIES IN ENGLISH MEDIEVAL LANGUAGE AND LITERATURE

Edited by Jacek Fisiak

Vol. 53

PETER LANG

Middle English Names of Medical Preparations

Marta Sylwanowicz

Middle English Names of Medical Preparations

Towards a Standard Medical Terminology

PETER LANG

Bibliographic Information published by the Deutsche Nationalbibliothek
The Deutsche Nationalbibliothek lists this publication in the Deutsche Nationalbibliografie; detailed bibliographic data is available in the internet at http://dnb.d-nb.de.

Library of Congress Cataloging-in-Publication Data
A CIP catalog record for this book has been applied for at the Library of Congress.

This publication was financially supported by
the University of Social Sciences, Warsaw.

ISSN 1436-7521
ISBN 978-3-631-74779-7 (Print)
E-ISBN 978-3-631-76001-7 (E-PDF)
E-ISBN 978-3-631-76002-4 (EPUB)
E-ISBN 978-3-631-76003-1 (MOBI)
DOI 10.3726/b14300

Peter Lang – Berlin · Bern · Bruxelles · New York ·
Oxford · Warszawa · Wien

This publication has been peer reviewed.

www.peterlang.com

Table of contents

List of tables

List of figures

Abbreviations

(a) Text corpus abbreviations

ACH	*Agnus Castus: A Middle English Herbal* (MS 10.90, Royal Library, Stockholm)
AFS	*Treatises of Fistula in Ano, Haemorrhoids, and Clysters* by John Arderne (MS Sloane 6, British Library, London)
AntN	*Antidotarium Nicholai* (MS Ferguson 147, University Library, Glasgow)
AW	*Alchemical Waters* (MS Harley 2381, British Library, London)
BG	*Benvenutus Grassus* (MS Hunter V.8.6, University Library, Glasgow)
BS	*Book of Surgery* (MS Harley 1736, British Library, London)
CExp	Cophon, *Experimentes* (MS Additional 34111, British Library, London)
CHIR	*Chirurgie de 1392* (MS 564, Wellcome Historical Medical Library, London)
CrophB	*Crophill's Books* (remedies) (MS Harley 1735, British Library, London)
DPP	*De caritate, þe priuyte of priuyteis* (MS Toshiyuki Takamiya 38, Tokyo)
FCC	*First Corpus Compendium* (MS Corp-C 388, Cambridge)
GA	*Gilbertus Anglicus* (MS 537, Wellcome Historical Medical Library, London)
GAC	*Gilbertus Anglicus, Compendium* (epilepsy) (MS 19079, Huntington Library, San Marino)
GCA1	Guy de Chauliac, *Anatomy* (MS 12, New York Academy of Medicine)
GCA2	Guy de Chauliac, *Anatomy* (MS 25, Biblioteque Nationale, Paris)
GCFD	Guy de Chauliac, *Treatise on Fractures and Dislocations* (MS 12, New York Academy of Medicine, New York)
GCM	Guy de Chauliac, *Chirurgia Magna* (MS 336/725, Gonville and Caius College, Cambridge)
GCU	Guy de Chauliac, *Treatise on Ulcers* (MS 12, New York Academy of Medicine, New York)

GCW	Guy de Chauliac, *Treatise on Wounds* (MS 12, New York Academy of Medicine, New York)
HMW	Henslow, *Medical Works of the Fourteenth Century* (MS Harley 2378; Sloane 2584; Sloane 521, British Libray, London)
HRec	Heinrich, *Recipes* (MS Additional 33996, British Library, London)
JBurg	John of Burgundy, *Plague Treatise* (MS Sloane 2320, British LIbrary, London)
LChP	Lanfranc, *Chirurgia Parva* (MS 397, Wellcome Medical Library, London)
LDM	*Liber de Diversis Medicinis* (MS Thornton A.5.2, Cathedral Library, Lincoln)
LeechB1	*Leechbook 1* (MS 136, Medical Society of London Library, London)
LeechB2	*Leechbook 2* (MS 405, Wellcome Medical Library, London)
LSC1	Lanfranc, *Sciencie of Cirurgie 1* (MS Ashmole 1396, Bodleian Library, Oxford)
LSC2	Lanfranc, *Sciencie of Cirurgie 2* (MS Additional 12056, British Library, London)
MedCh	*Medical Charms* (MS Additional 34111, British Library, London)
MedW	*Medical Works* (MS Harley 2378; Sloane 2584; Sloane 521, British Library, London)
QE	*Quintessence* (MS Sloane 73, British Library, London)
REC	*Recipes* (MS Hunter 185, Glasgow University Library)
RS	*Regimen sanitatis* (MS Rawlinson C.83, Bodleian Library, Oxford)
RupQ	John of Rupescissa, *Quintessence* (MS Ferguson 205, University Library, Glasgow)
RupR	John of Rupescissa, *Remedies* (MS Ferguson 205, University Library, Glasgow)
SCC	*Second Corpus Compendium* (MS Corp-C 388, Cambridge)
SW1	*Sekenesse of wymmen 1* (MS 47, Medical Library, Yale)
SW2	*Sekenesse of wymmen 2* (MS Sloane 2463, British Library, London)
ThP	*Thesaurus Pauperum* (MS Sloane 3489, British Library, London)
TTP	Torrella, *Tretece of the Pokkis* (MS Sloane 389, British Library, London)

WBMP	*Wyse Book od Maystyr Peers of Salerne* (MS Med. Misc. I, No. 3, College of Physicians of Philadelphia)

(b) Dictionaries

AND	Anglo-Norman Dictionary
BT	Bosworth-Toller's Anglo-Saxon Dictionary
CED	Collins English Dictionary
DMD	Dorland's Medical Dictionary
DMLBS	Dictionary of Medieval Latin from British Sources
DMVE	Dictionary of Medical Vocabulary in English, 1375–1550
DOE	Dictionary of Old English
DOEC	Dictionary of Old English Corpus
HTE	Historical Thesaurus of English
MED	Middle English Dictionary
OED	Oxford English Dictionary
TOE	Thesaurus of Old English

(c) Language abbreviations

Ar.	Arabic
AN	Anglo-Norman
CL	Classical Latin
Eng.	English
Fr.	French
Gmc	Germanic
Gk	Greek
L	Latin
ME	Middle English
MF	Middle French
ML	Medieval Latin
OE	Old English
OF	Old French

(d) Other

adj.	adjective
c.	century
cf.	compare
e.g.	exempli gratia/for example

etc.	et cetera
Fig.	Figure
ger.	gerund
i.e.	id est/that is
MEMT	Middle English Medical Texts
MS(S)	manuscript(s)
n.	noun
PDE	Present-Day English
pref.	prefix
Rem.	remedy books
RNF	relative normalized frequency
Spec.	specialised treatises
suf.	suffix
Surg.	surgical works
v.	verb

Preface and acknowledgements

Middle English medical lexicon has attracted various degrees of attention. Although some works offer a thorough examination and overview of a number of lexical fields, e.g. names of sicknesses or body parts, there are still areas that require intensive research. The present study aims to provide a comprehensive examination of Middle English names of pharmaceutical preparations. Particular attention will be given to the classification of the terms, their origin, structure and their distribution in Middle English medical writings.

The first two chapters serve as a theoretical background for the present study. Chapter one offers an overview of previous research on Middle English vocabularies, especially medical terminologies. This is followed by a presentation of the approach taken in the study and the description of medical texts examined for the present work. Chapter two contains a brief account of the development of pharmacy and medicine in medieval Europe and England. Chapters three to five contain the analyses of the collected material, with reference to terms relating to medical preparations found in the examined sources.

For practical purposes, the material has been divided into three groups: general names denoting a medical preparation (e.g. *medicine*, *remedy*), names denoting dosage forms (e.g. *ointment*, *pill*, *powder*, *syrup*), and names denoting specifics (e.g. *apostolicon*, *black powder of Arnald*, *emplaster dissolutive*, *mithridatum*, *red ointment*, *unguentum viridum*).

I wish to extend my thanks to all those who have helped me in preparing this book. First of all, I would like to thank Professor Jerzy Wełna for his inspiration in pursuing my studies, and for his valuable comments and suggestions that let this work see fruition. While writing this work I have been fortunate to enjoy the support of my colleagues, Magdalena Bator, D.Litt. and Anna Wojtyś, D.Litt., who have been exceptionally generous with their time and have patiently answered questions concerning the shape of the present work. Finally, I would like to thank my friends and family for their encouragement and understanding. My greatest debt is to my mother who has always believed in me and who has motivated me at every stage in the preparation of this work.

Chapter one: A review of previous research and an outline of the present study

1.1 Introduction

The present chapter opens with a short survey of the early research on Middle English lexicon, with focus on the studies of medical terminologies. The sections that follow contain a statement of the study purpose and the principles of approach to the analysis of the data. The last section provides a description of the text corpus.

1.2 Earlier studies on the lexicon of Middle English

The examination of Middle English lexis has attracted attention of so many scholars that a full account of the relevant monographs would require a separate publication[1]. Therefore, due to limitation of space, only a number of studies will be referred to below. Particular attention will be given to works published in the last three decades, though references to some earlier texts that may have laid solid foundations for later studies will also be made. An account of general studies on the development of Middle English lexis is followed by an outline description of works on various lexical fields, with a focus on contributions to the study of Middle English medical terminology.

Middle English lexicon is dealt with in most studies on the history and development of the English language (e.g. Jespersen 1972 [1905], Strang 1970, Baugh — Cable 1978, Blake 1992, Millward 1996, Fisiak 2000, Fennel 2001, Pyles — Algeo 2004, Crystal 2006, Hogg — Denison 2008, Algeo — Butcher 2013). These works,

1 Anyone interested in the historical studies on the English lexicon can start with consulting detailed bibliographies of earlier research on the English language. There is a monumental work by Kennedy (1927), who offers an index of language studies produced since the beginning of printing till 1922. Later publications continued the work of Kennedy by updating the bibliography, e.g., Müller-Schwefe (1962), Oizumi (1966), Kohl (1970), Fisiak (1977, 1983), Tajima (1988), etc. There is also an online database of works (ABELL - *Annual Bibliography of English Language and Literature*) from 1892 till today, which is updated monthly. Most of these sources cover all language areas, but there are also reference books dedicated to the word studies, e.g., Cameron et al. (1983), or Sylvester — Robert's (2000) bibliographies of studies on Old and Middle English lexicon, respectively. In the latter, apart from a mere list of works there is a short note about their content.

however, contain relatively brief sections on the vocabularies of particular historical periods. More detailed discussions can be found in studies on the development of the English lexicon, such as Serjeantson (1935), Hughes (1988, 2000), Minkova — Stockwell (2009), Miller (2012), Durkin (2014), etc.

In addition to the diachronic studies of English lexis, a large number of contributions are exclusively devoted to the Middle English period. Many such works concentrate on foreign influences (e.g. Baugh 1935, Prins 1941–1942, Rothwell 1980, 1998, Dekeyser 1991, Dance 2003, Bator 2006, 2010, 2015, Krygier 2012), or on the rivalry between particular lexical items (e.g. Rynell 1948, Ogura 1981, 2005, Dekeyser 1995, Sylwanowicz 2003, 2007, Wełna 2005, 2009, Sądej 2007, Sądej-Sobolewska 2011a,b, 2012, Kłos 2010, Esquibel — Wojtyś 2012, Bator 2013a,b, 2015, Esquibel 2015, Molencki 2015, 2018).

The examination of the Middle English lexicon has also resulted in a large number of lexico-semantic studies. Several contributions concentrate on references to people (e.g. Kjellmer 1973, Diensberg 1985, Kleparski 1997, 2005, Grygiel 2008, Bator 2009a, Ciszek 2013), while other deal with various aspects of personal life, e.g. lexis of sex (Coleman 1996), personal hygiene (Sądej-Sobolewska — Sylwanowicz 2011), or cloth and clothing (Chambers 2009, Chambers — Owen-Crocker 2008, Chambers — Sylvester 2010a,b,c, Sylvester 2012, Sylvester et al. 2014, Chambers 2017)[2]. Here, we cannot miss works devoted to the investigation of terms concerning more abstract ideas like human emotions (e.g. Diller 1996, 2011, Sylvester 2000, Fabiszak 2001, Ogura 2013, Miura 2015), human senses (e.g. Bator 2009b, 2012), the concepts of "chance" and "fortune" (e.g. Bately 1996), or "clean" and "dirt" (e.g. Markus 2008, Sylwanowicz 2012), etc.

Other works contain accounts of the vocabularies of fauna and flora in Middle English. The former concentrate on the names of beasts from the real world (e.g. Filipowicz 2010, Dyke 2012, Scott-Macnab 2013, 2014, Sauer — Scott-Macnab 2017) and the realms of fantasy (e.g. Karczmarczyk 2011, 2012), or on metaphorical extensions of terms referring to domesticated animals (e.g. Kiełtyka 2008). The flora works deal with the names of plants (e.g. Hunt 1989, Wallner 1992, Norri 1996, Sauer 1996, 2011).

Many scholars have turned their attention to the terms relating to law and crime (e.g. Olszewska 1935, Bately 2000, Roberts 2000), hunting (e.g. Savage 1951, Scott-Macnab 2003), religion (e.g. Newman 2006, Łodej 2012), seafaring (e.g. Sandahl

2 These works are an outcome of the project *The Lexis of Cloth and Clothing in Britain c. 700–1450: Origins, Identification, Contexts and Change* hosted by the University of Manchester. For more on the project see: http://lexisproject.arts.manchester.ac.uk/research/index.html (date of last access: September 2017).

1951, 1959, 1982, Sayers 1998), names of occupations (e.g. Thuresson 1950, Mills 1968, Dobrovolska 2017), settlements (Svensson 1997, Svensson — Hering 2010), technology and administration (Crespo García — Moskowich Spiegel 2004), or culinary practice (e.g. Serjeantson 1938, Carroll 1997, Frantzen 2011, Kornexl — Lenker 2011, Bator 2011, 2012, 2013a,b,c, 2014, Rusinek 2013, or Bator — Sylwanowicz 2016, 2017a)[3].

Although Middle English can also boast of texts that deal with popular and practical science, such as astrology, prognostication, horticulture, medicine, etc. (cf. Matheson 1994)[4], that offer valuable materials for a linguistic investigation, the majority of studies have focused on the examination of medical writings.

One of the earliest works on Middle English medical vocabularies is Schöffler's (1919) alphabetical list of Middle English medical terms unattested or inadequately explained in the *New English Dictionary*, the forerunner of the *Oxford English Dictionary* (OED). Wallner (1964b, 1971, 1976) lists words not recorded in OED, while Norri (1987) examines medical vocabulary (names of sicknesses, parts of the body, medicinal substances) in four remedy books written around the middle of the 15th century. In his later works Norri (1992, 1998) provides a more comprehensive linguistic analysis of the names of sicknesses and of body parts recorded in the medical texts dating from the 15th and the first half of the 16th century. These findings are summarised in Norri (2004), who concentrates on exits and entrances in English medical vocabulary. Further studies on medical word-stock were undertaken by Sylwanowicz (2006, 2007) who examined the medieval terminology of mental diseases, focusing on the use and distribution of two terms: *madness* and *insanity.* In her later works, Sylwanowicz (2009, 2011, 2014a,b, 2015) provided a survey of the names of medieval surgical instruments, examined the semantic development of medieval synonyms of *sickness*-nouns, and finally turned her attention to the names of pharmaceutical preparations[5].

---

3 The last two studies (Bator — Sylwanowicz 2016, 2017a) are part of a series of publications devoted to *The Synchronic and Diachronic Comparative Analysis of the Culinary and Medical Recipes in the History of English*, a three-year project financed by the National Science Centre in Poland (OPUS 6).

4 For a comprehensive history of science in medieval times see, e.g., Lindberg — Shank (2015).

5 Apart from the studies on terminology, a number of works concentrate on translation techniques (e.g. Voigts — McVaugh 1984, Minnis 1987, Wallner 1987, Jones 1989 or Pahta 1998) and on strategies used in the process of vernacularization of medical treatises (articles in Taavitsainen — Pahta 2004). There are also studies devoted to the

The above brief survey of the works that deal with various terminologies shows that the lexicon of Middle English seems to be an "unexhausted mine", and there is still much work to be done and many lexical fields to be explored.

1.3 Purpose of the study

A number of earlier scholars studying the history of English scientific and medical terminology often maintained that the major developments in English scientific lexicon took place from the 16th century onwards (e.g. Schäfer 1989, Görlach 1993, Knowles 1997). Earlier English, as Schäfer (1989: 1) claims, "was incapable of providing a linguistic medium for traditional scholarship, and for the rapidly developing scientific disciplines, since it lacked the necessary terminologies". This dismissive view of any pre-1500 progress in the evolution of scientific terminology was challenged by, e.g., McConchie's (1997) results of the examination of vocabulary in medical works published between 1547 and 1612. The author demonstrates that the medical lexicon of the 16th century owes much to the developments in the medical vocabularies of the earlier periods. This finding is confirmed by, e.g., Norri's (1992) or Sylwanowicz's (2014a) thorough examinations of Middle English names of sicknesses.

The present monograph, yet another contribution to the study of early English scientific vocabularies, will reveal that Middle English laid solid foundation for the development of medical terminologies. Its main aim is to offer a systematic and comprehensive examination of the names of medical preparations used in the 14th–15th century medical writings. The emphasis will be put on the origin of the terms, their structure, as well as their distribution and presentation in texts representing different traditions of medical writing.

The choice of the period to be examined, i.e. 14th–15th centuries, is conditioned by the available sources. For instance, the MEMT corpus, consisting of the largest selection of Middle English medical writings (the total of half-a-million words), includes texts produced around 1330, and between c. 1375 and c. 1500.

medical recipe (e.g. Jones 1998a, Alonso Almeida 1999, Taavitsainen 2001, Mäkinen 2004, 2006, Quintana-Toledo 2009, Bator — Sylwanowicz 2017a,b,c, Sylwanowicz 2017a,b, Cruz-Cabanillas 2017).

1.4 Names of medicines: classification and methods of analysis[6]

Compiling a corpus and selecting a method to study the names of medical preparations was a starting point of this work. The first step was to make a list of all Middle English references to 'any substance or preparation used in the treatment of disease' (OED, *medicine* n.[1]). This involved listing names of medicines from various dictionaries, glossaries, etc., and browsing the Middle English medical writings to find all the instances and possible variants of the names of medicines and items not listed in the dictionaries.

At this point the question of delimitation arose: which items should be included in the lexical field of medicines? Medieval medications were often classified as simple and compound medicines[7]; where the first group contained preparations made of one herb only, while the second was composed of several ingredients. The inclusion of herb terminology would greatly increase the size of the corpus, which would require a separate study. Moreover, since much has already been done in the field of medieval names of herbs and plants (cf. the references listed in section 1.2), the present work is restricted to the analysis of compound medicines understood here as 'compositions of at least two elements'[8].

However, other difficulties concerning the inclusion of particular lexical items have been encountered. As observed by Norri (1992: 89, 2004: 106) in his analysis of the lexical fields of Middle English names of sicknesses and body parts, most discussions of lexical fields concentrate on single words and exclude compounds and phrases from their analysis. This understanding of a lexical field would restrict the analysis to general names (e.g. *medicine, remedy, antidote)* or selected names for specifics (e.g. *apostolicon*, *marciaton*, *triacle*, etc.) and exclude combinations

---

6 A preliminary classification of the names of medical preparations and the discussion of possible problems with their identification have been proposed by Sylwanowicz (2015). The material has been extended and thoroughly revised for the purposes of the present study. Possible differences between the article and the present work are partly due to the differences in the corpora used then and now.

7 For more on the division into simple and compound medicines see section 2.7 in chapter two.

8 Following Norri (2016), the exception has been made with regard to the names of oils and waters which, according to medieval classification were treated as simple medicines, i.e. 'preparations composed of one ingredient'. As Norri (2016: 4) explains, "[it] was not always possible to determine the exact ingredients of a medicinal oil or water from the context, and in some cases to include or exclude according to difference between simple and compound would have been somewhat arbitrary".

such as *unguentum album*, *unguentum viride*, *ointment resolutive*, *drying plaster*, *emplastrum Gratia Dei*, *Rhazes' white plaster* or *syrup of horehound*, all of which are found in various medical recipes. Therefore, for the purposes of this study, Lipka's understanding of the concept of the lexical field has been adopted. Lipka (1992: 152) proposes a distinction between a "word-field", "exclusively including morphologically simple items", and a "lexical field", "consisting of simple and complex lexemes". Thus, combinations listed above are also included in the lexical field of medicines.

The next issue that had to be considered while collecting the names of medicines was that of inclusion or exclusion of terms of foreign origin. The question to be answered was which term could be regarded as an established part of English medical terminology. The material reveals that the same compiler who translates a text with varying degrees of freedom, is often inconsistent in the use of terms. For instance, the compiler of the *Wyse Book of Maystyr Peers of Salerne* (MEMT, 15th c. *WBMP* (MS Med. Misc. I)) uses Latin names of medicines in the headings of each recipe and then repeats the name by giving its equivalent in English (1ab). However, occasionally the translator repeats the Latin term instead of adducing native terms (1cd), cf.:

(1) a. To make **vnguentum viridum**. ffor to make **a grene oynement**. (MEMT, 15th c. *WBMP* (MS Med. Misc. I), 312)
b. **Emplastrum Oxiorociu**. Also here be the makyng of playstrys, and fyrste to make yis **plastyr Oxiorocin**. (MEMT, 15th c. *WBMP* (MS Med. Misc. I), 314)
c. **Emplastyr Jerusalem**. Also for to make thys **Emplaystyr Jerusalem**. (MEMT, 15th c. *WBMP* (MS Med. Misc. I), 314),
d. **Vnguentum salsum**. Also for to make thys oynment **vnguentum Salsum**. (MEMT, 15th c. *WBMP* (MS Med. Misc. I), 313)

Sometimes the compiler retains the Latin term followed by a description of how to prepare the medicine and instructions which sickness could be cured with the use of this medicine, cf.:

(2) **ffor Grene Entrette**. Take Bugle, Pygle, Senegle, Betayn, Anens, smallache Croppes of the rede brere (…). (MEMT, 15th c. *WBMP* (MS Med. Misc. I), 310)

In addition, in various texts one often comes across instances where two Latin forms of the same term occur, e.g., *vnguentum arabicum - vnguento arabico*. The question that arises in such cases is which one is an accepted "English" form of a Latin technical term? In this case, the Middle English translation of Guy de Chauliac's surgery (Ogden 1971: 290, after Norri 2004: 107) is of much help. The author of the translation explains that Latin forms in the nominative are accepted "English" terms, cf.:

(3) Afterward clense it wiþ vnguentum apostolorum (It myghte be saide wiþ vnguento apostolorum in þis translacioun, and þat were more sewynge the fourme and congruyte of gramer, but alle suche termes of Latyn schal be schewed in þis Englisshynge in þe nomynatyf case, for-why þe Latyn of þe nominatyf case is most vsed among Englisshe termes. And also it is so beste to be vndersonden in commune langage, and most esy, namely to men þat can but þe comune langage.) or wiþ vnguentum Egipcianum.

Another difficulty is posed by terms which are attested in only one medical treatise. Here, the criterion of frequency of occurrence might be the solution when deciding about the exclusion of the term from the lexicon. However, a term's very low frequency of use need not mean that it was not an element of the Middle English medical lexicon. In addition, there still remain many texts which have not been edited or studied, and one is never certain which items were common or rare.

Considering the above, all names denoting 'a preparation used in the treatment of illness' and occurring in an English context are collected and listed in the corpus. The only exception are Latin forms other than nominative (cf. also Norri 2004: 107).

Once the list of medicines was completed, another question arose, i.e. how to classify these items to ensure a clear and comprehensible analysis of the material. One possibility is to group them regarding the conditions they are aimed to cure or according to the body parts affected by a disorder. However, while reading through medical texts one learns that a single medicinal substance is meant to heal various ailments and body parts, cf.:

(4) PIGRA GALIENI (…). Yt ys good for **al ache of þe hed** of coldnes, **of þe stomake**, yt strayneþ vomyte; yt helpeþ moche **to coldnes of þe matrice**; yt helpeþ conseyuynge. (MEMT, 15th c. *AntN* (MS Ferguson 147), f. 37r)
TIRICATA MAGNA (…). Yt ys goode for þe greuosseste yuelis of al þe body. Yt ys good **for þe faldynge yuel, þe swonyng yuel**, and **for þe migrayme.** (MEMT, 15th c. *AntN* (MS Ferguson 147), f. 43v)
UNGUENTUM MARCEATOUN (…). Yt ys goode **for ache of þe hed**, and **for coldnes of þe stomak, of þe splene, and of þe lyuer**. (MEMT, 15th c. *AntN* (MS Ferguson 147), f. 51v)

Thus, according to the suggested classification many names would be repeated in different categories. All the three medicines under (4) could be categorised as serving to cure the ailments of the head, while *pigra galieni* and *unguentum marceatoun* could also be considered as medicines healing the ailments of the stomach. Examples like *tricata magna*, on the other hand, announce further problems with assigning the right category: should *faldynge yuel* 'epilepsy', *swonyng yuel* 'swooning, fainting or noise in the ears' and *migrayme* 'severe headache, migraine' be treated as representing the ailments of the head or as two or three different conditions? For instance, present-day medicine explains epilepsy as a neurological problem, whereas in the Middle Ages there dominated a view that a person suffering from epilepsy was possessed by some evil power. Even if a more scholarly explanation was offered by medical authorities, we learn from them that it was often difficult to identify the source of epileptic convulsions. Although Galen claimed that brain was partly responsible for the convulsions, others explained that epilepsy was due to the excess of phlegm in the blood, too much blood in veins, distress or lack of food or sex (cf. Chaudhary et al. 2011). The fact that medieval knowledge about and understanding of various bodily disorders differed much from what we know today is another factor that reveals the weaknesses of the above classification.

The second possible way of classifying the material is to group the material according to the origin of each lexeme (e.g. Germanic, Latin or French). This approach is also problematic as there are such examples as *balm - salve - ointment - unguent*, *plaster - emplaster*, *powder - puluer*, or *oil of roses - oleum rosarum*. In each group or pair lexical items share the meaning but differ in their provenance. Thus, discussing them on the basis of their origin would mean that synonymous items would end up in separate sections.

An alternative solution, though not free of shortcomings, would be to divide references to medical substances into three large categories: (i) general terms denoting medical preparations, (ii) terms denoting dosage forms, and (iii) terms denoting specifics. A careful reading of various medical texts has revealed that most of the terms considered in this study could be identified as representative of one of the above-mentioned categories. Such division allows one to observe the rivalry between items related by meaning or form, but of different etymology.

The last and the largest group of words and expressions, i.e. names denoting specifics, apart from single words, contains also complex forms. Therefore, for practical reasons, the material has been split into two large categories: (i) simplex[9] terms and derivatives and (ii) compounds and phrases. The first group includes simplex forms together with derivatives because of problems with determining whether the examined words (e.g. forms with the suffix *-tion*, such as *digestion*, *fomentation*, *purgation*) were direct loans from French or Latin, subsequently treated as simplex forms, or English formations "on a Neo-Latin basis" (Marchand 1969: 216) in which it would be possible to identify allomorphs of

9 The term *simplex* has been adopted after Bauer (2002: 29–30) who uses it with reference to words not divisible into smaller parts (cf. also Norri 1992: 90).

English morphemes (cf. Middle English verbs *digesten, fomenten, purgen*). Other problematic forms are nouns with the suffix *-er* which might be either derivatives with Eng. *-er* or adoptions of forms with Fr. *-(i)er(e)*.

As regards compounds and phrases, they are treated cumulatively as there is no clear distinction between the two formations, at least in Middle English texts. According to various sources (e.g. Marchand 1969, Adams 1982, Lipka 1992, Bauer 2002), criteria such as stress pattern or spelling might be helpful in identifying compounds. However, "all of them are of limited value and neither singly nor in combination are they sufficient to decide all doubtful cases". (Sauer 1992: 714). For instance, having access to written sources only, it is hardly possible to verify how words were actually stressed in medieval texts. Sauer (1992: 714) adds that even texts in verse are not helpful as "the verse accent can override the (presumed) normal accent pattern". Similarly, inconsistent variant forms of compounds (sometimes spaced, sometimes hyphenated or printed as one word) make spelling an unreliable criterion. As a result, it was found appropriate to discuss compounds together with phrases, i.e. "word-groups used as words" (Leisi — Mair 1999: § 16) that were used as names (cf. Marchand 1969: 122–127, Koziol 1972, 69ff., Sauer — Scott-Macnab 2017: 188).

The full list of the names of medicaments examined for the present study is to be found in the Appendices. Appendix A lists general terms denoting medical preparations and those denoting dosage forms, both groups being discussed in chapters three and four respectively. Appendix B includes the largest group of lexical items, i.e. terms denoting specifics. They are grouped according to the division proposed in chapter five, i.e. two main categories based on word formation patterns, which are further divided into semantic groups. For details concerning their division, see chapter five and the introductory remarks in Appendix B.

1.5 Corpus texts and editorial principles

The material examined for the present work consists of medical writings included in the *Middle English Medical Texts* (MEMT), an electronic corpus containing texts from c. 1375–1500. The corpus divides the texts into three main categories: surgical treatises, specialised texts, and remedy books (Taavitsainen — Pahta — Mäkinen 2005)[10]. Apart from the major categories of texts, the MEMT corpus contains also two collections (*First corpus compendium* and

10 For a more detailed discussion of the division of Middle English medical texts see section 2.5 in chapter two.

Second corpus compendium) written in the first half of the 14th century, which are included in the Appendix section to the MEMT corpus. These texts represent the remedy book tradition.

The MEMT corpus, with some exceptions, includes only fragments of texts. Therefore, the material for the present study has been supplemented with the full versions of the following works:

Surgical treatises:

- two English translations of Guido Lanfranc's *Science of Cirurgie* (Fleischhacker 1894) edited from:
  - MS Ashmole 1396, Bodleian Library, Oxford;
  - MS Additional 12056, British Library, London;
- two English translations of Guy de Chauliac's *Anatomy* (Wallner 1964a) edited from:
  - MS 12, New York Academy of Medicine;
  - MS 25, Biblioteque Nationale, Paris;
- Guy de Chauliac's *Treatise on Fractures and Dislocations* (Wallner 1969) edited from MS 12, New York Academy of Medicine, New York;
- Guy de Chauliac's *Chirurgia Magna* (Wallner 1971) edited from MS 336/725, Gonville and Caius College, Cambridge;
- Guy de Chauliac's *Treatise on Wounds* (Wallner 1976) edited from MS 12, New York Academy of Medicine, New York;
- Guy de Chauliac's *Treatise on Ulcers* (Wallner 1982) edited from MS 12, New York Academy of Medicine, New York;
- John Arderne's *Treatises of Fistula in Ano, Haemorrhoids, and Clysters* (Power 1910) edited from MS Sloane 6, British Library, London.

Specialised texts:

- *The Sekenesse of Wymmen* (Hallaert 1982) edited from MS 47, Medical Library, Yale;
- *Medieval Woman's Guide to Health* (Rowland 1981) edited from MS Sloane 2463, British Library, London.

Remedy books:

- *Healing and Society in Medieval England: A Middle English Translation of the Pharmaceutical Writings of Gilbertus Anglicus* (Getz 1991) edited from MS 537, Wellcome Historical Medical Library, London;
- *A Middle English Medical Remedy Book* (Alonso Almeida 2014) edited from MS Hunter 185, Glasgow University Library.

In order to make the list of references to medical preparations as comprehensive as possible and to verify the date of their occurrence, their sense or their etymology, a number of dictionaries have been consulted. These include the online editions of:

- *Anglo-Norman Dictionary* (http://www.anglo-norman.net);
- Bosworth — Toller's *Anglo-Saxon Dictionary* (http://bosworth.ff.cuni.cz);
- *Dictionary of Medieval Latin from British Sources* (http://www.dmlbs.ox.ac.uk);
- *Dorland's Medical Dictionary* (https://dorlandsonline.com);
- *Historical Thesaurus of English* (www.oed.com/thesaurus);
- *Middle English Dictionary* (https://quod.lib.umich.edu/m/med/);
- *Oxford English Dictionary* (www.oed.com);

as well as:

- *A Thesaurus of Old English* (Roberts et al. 2000);
- *Dictionary of Medical Vocabulary in English, 1375–1550* (Norri 2016);
- *Dictionary of Old English* (diPaolo Healey et al. 2008);
- *Medical Meanings. A Glossary of Word Origins* (Haubrich 1997).

Due to the fact that some of the analysed terms had a medical meaning already in Old English, the earliest English medical sources have also been examined. These include the following text editions:

- *Leechdoms, Wortcunning and Starcraft of Early England* (Cockayne 1864–1866), including the 10th c. *Leechbook* - a collection of medical writings translated from Latin – and divided into three books: Book I and Book II (Bald's *Leechbook*), and Book III (*Leechbook* III);
- *Lacnunga*, a collection randomly compiled by non-medical scribes, dealing mostly with folk medicine (Cockayne 1864–1866);
- *The Old English Herbarium and Medicina de Quadrupedibus* (Vriend 1984), the Old English translations of Latin descriptions of herbs and plants, and their curative properties.

A large number of sources and a variety of ways they offer in providing information about extracts from manuscripts or book editions, required an introduction of some uniform editorial conventions. All quotations used in the present study preserve the format introduced in the corpora, including capitalizations and punctuation. As regards information about the source, the description of examples starts with an abbreviated title of the main source (in the case of MEMT and dictionaries) or the name of the editor (in the case of edited writings). This is followed by a date of the manuscript, short title of a text, and information about the manuscript, as derived from *Middle English Dictionary Compendium HyperBibliography*. The final element consists of references to specific pages, lines or folios. In the references to edited manuscripts the page number of the edition is given, followed by the information on where the line begins and ends. In other cases, references follow the conventions introduced by the sources. The following examples illustrate the above editorial principles:

- for dictionaries and MEMT:
  (DMVE, a1425 *Arderne(3)* (MS Em 69), 177r)
  (MED,?a1425 **Chauliac(1)* (MS NY 12), 139a/a)
  (MEMT, 15th c. *AntN* (MS Ferguson 147), f. 6r)
- for edited works:
  (Fleischhacker, a1400 *LSC1* (MS Ashm 1396), 17/10)
  (Getz, a1475 *GA* (MS Wel 537), 152/6–8)
  (Wallner, 1425 *GCA1* (MS NY 12), 26/10–11)

As regards the presentation of references to medical preparations, which have been recorded with many spelling variants, I have adopted the strategy applied by the editor of the *Dictionary of Medical Vocabulary in English, 1375–1550,* i.e. (i) only the commonest spelling variant is given (for all the variants the DMVE, MED, OED, MEMT and text editions can be consulted), (ii) if the medieval form is close to the corresponding Present-day English term, the modern form is given (e.g. ME *plaester, plaestre, plaister, playster*, etc. are rendered as *plaster*), (iii) terms adopted from Latin are adduced in their original form (e.g. *oleum*, *unguentum*).

Chapter two: Medieval English medicine and pharmacy

2.1 Introduction

Pharmacy, i.e. preparation and use of medicines, is one of those occupations that existed long before recorded history. Hence, it is difficult to determine when and how the first therapeutic substances were discovered and compounded. As Porter (2001: 246) observes: "Bitter experience taught people which plants were toxic, and, happier events perhaps suggested, more subtly, that some had beneficial properties". However, it is known from various records that the earliest medical preparations, mostly from materia medica of animal, vegetable and mineral sources, were used by a number of ancient civilizations that developed complex levels of medical knowledge and laid solid foundations for the development of pharmaceutical and medical practice (Anderson 2005, Marriott et al. 2010).

Before examining the medical records, it is essential to become familiarized with the medical theory, nature of pharmacy and actual practice that prevailed at the time. Because pharmacy and medicine were practically inseparable in their early history (Anderson 2005: 5), both areas will be taken into account in the following discussion. The general characteristics of medicine and pharmacy and the society in which both occupations were practiced should allow one to understand fully the nature (i.e. meanings, connotations and use) of the terms studied for this work.

This chapter, containing a brief historical account of the development of pharmacy and medical practice, which begins with the presentation of the origins of medicines making and healing practices, provides a theoretical and social background of medieval English medicine and pharmacy. It also contains a brief account of people's involvement in medical practice, their social position and conditions in which they worked. This is followed by an overview of English major medical works and a classification of the products of pharmacy.

2.2 Origins of medicine and pharmacy

The earliest known traces of medical and pharmaceutical practice go back to the cultures of Mesopotamia, in particular the Sumerians (3000–2400 BC), who are believed to have used plant drugs, wound washings, plasters and bandaging (Anderson 2005). At the same time, another influential civilization was emerging: the Egyptians. That their medical knowledge was much more advanced, we can learn from papyrus scrolls, found in caves and tombs. One such document, *The Papyrus Ebers*[11], which resembles in its form a modern collection of recipes, contains about 875 prescriptions and a list of 700 drugs, many of which are still in use today. Although magic and sorcery were present in medical practice, the Egyptians tended to turn to more scientific methods of healing. It is also believed that one of the well-known pharmacy symbols, the *Rx* sign, which is nowadays found as a heading in most medical prescriptions, is probably derived from the Egyptian eye symbol: "the eye of Horus, the god of the sun, often represented as a falcon or a man with the head of falcon" (Taylor 2008: 108). According to another, more often quoted, interpretation, *Rx* stands for L *recipere* 'take', an abbreviation found in many Latin medical recipes. The English word *recipe* 'a list of ingredients and instructions for preparing something, usually a dish' is derived from a Latin form (Taylor 2008, Bator — Sylwanowicz 2016).

The two civilizations, those of Mesopotamia and Egypt, had a great influence on the development of Greek medicine (1250–285 BC), which made use of "three sources of knowledge: the temple practice of Asclepius or healing by the gods; the physiological opinions of philosophers; and the practice of superintendents of the gymnasia" (Anderson 2005: 27). The Rod of Asclepius, a serpent-entwined staff, became the official symbol of medicine and health care. Although there are many interpretations of the symbolic meaning of the serpent and the rod, most overlap with the one given by Cornutus, a Greek philosopher (active in the 1st century AD), who in his *Theologiae Graece Compendium* offers the following explanation (Edelstein — Edelstein 1998: 13):

> Asclepius derived his name from healing soothingly and from deferring the withering that comes with death. For this reason, therefore, they give him a serpent as an attribute, indicating that those who avail themselves of medical science undergo a process similar to the serpent in that they, as it were, grow young again after illnesses and slough off old age; also because the serpent is a sign of attention, much of which is required in medical treatments. The staff also seems to be a symbol of some similar thing. For by means of this it is set before our minds that unless we are supported by such inventions as these, in so far as falling continually into sickness is concerned, stumbling along we would fall even sooner than necessary.

A similar symbol is a depiction of a serpent reaching up to touch the bowl (Hygeia's bowl), which represents a symbolic merger of medicine and pharmacy. Hygeia, one of the daughters of Asclepius, was the goddess of health, cleanliness and sanitation. In ancient Greece and Rome, all offerings to the goddess of health

11 For more on the *Papyrus Ebers* see, e.g., Gerald (2013: 28), Zebroski (2016: 24–25).

were given in a bowl or a patera (hence Hygeia's bowl), a vessel in which medicinal herbs were compounded. Therefore, today many pharmacy organisations use the bowl and the serpent as their symbol (Gasbarro 2005: 1–2).

Greek medicine did not solely rely on deities, and works of many philosophers, such as Hippocrates, Socrates, Plato and Aristotle, allowed medical practice to escape from the power of the supernatural (Anderson 2005, Taylor — Harding 2005). Hippocrates (460–377 BC) is considered one of the most revered Greek philosophers that introduced a more learned approach to health treatment. He is believed to have attempted to explain the natural causes and effects of sicknesses and produced descriptions of many ailments and epidemics, all contained in the *Hippocratic Corpus* written between 420 and 370 BC (Porter 2001: 58). Hippocratic medicine, as shown in the *Corpus*, relied heavily on a belief that a person's health was dependent upon keeping a balance of bodily fluids, i.e. humours. These humours were a direct reflection of the view that the world was made of four elements: air, fire, water and earth. The four elements were "generated through a combination of the four qualities, hot, cold, dry and moist: earth was cold and dry, air hot and moist, fire hot and dry, while water was cold and moist. The human body was regarded as a microcosm, and therefore man too was supposed to consist of four elements called humours. These were: blood (hot and moist), phlegm (cold and moist), yellow bile called choler (hot and dry), and black bile called melancholy (cold and dry). The balance resulting from the mixture of the elements in each individual determined a person's complexion" (Norri 1992: 41). If these humours (and elements) were in balance within the body, the body was healthy. But if the body became unbalanced, illness would result.

The premises of humoral theory and Greek medicine, as a whole, were later adopted by Roman scholars and physicians, whose medical knowledge and practice was quickly spread throughout Europe. To the most influential personalities of Roman medicine belonged Dioscorides (50–100 AD), the author of *Materia Medica* (a comprehensive list of materials of animal, plant and mineral origin with medicinal uses), and Galen of Pergamon (129–216 AD), a flourishing author of many medical theories that remained alive until the 17th century (Pahta — Taavitsainen 1995, Anderson 2005). Galen supported the Hyppocratic theory of the four fluids and combined it with the Pythagorean four elements (fire, air, earth, water) and the four temperaments of man: choleric, sanguine, melancholic, phlegmatic (Porter 2001: 58, Anderson 2005: 30–31).

Greek and Roman medical heritage became the basis of Arab medicine (400–1100 AD), whose practitioners copied and preserved the original Greek and Latin works and supplemented them with their own passages. Hunain ibn

Ishaq (809–873), Ar-Razi (latinized as Rhazes or Rasis, 865–925 AD) and Ibn Sina (or Avicenna, 980–1037 AD) are the major medical figures that often contributed to the expansion of Arab medical writing, knowledge and practice. Ibn Ishaq translated most works of Galen and "provided the Arabic world with more Galenic texts than survive today in their original Greek" (Porter 2001: 67). Rhazes published a medical compendium based on Greek, Syriac, Arabic, Persian and Indian sources, which he supplemented with his own observations on medical practice. He is also known for his pioneering chemical experiments. Avicenna, often called "the Hippocrates of the Arab world", is the author of *al Quanum* (the *Canon of Medicine*), which in the 12th century was translated into Latin and became the basis of medical studies for centuries. Today, the Royal Pharmaceutical Society of Great Britain has Avicenna and Galen in their coat of arms (Anderson 2005: 35).

The foundations of the Graeco-Roman and Arab medicine were quickly transferred to Western Europe. However, with the disintegration of the Roman Empire in the mid 4th century AD (Rome controlled the West and Constantinople the East) and the rising influence of Christianity, the Western world entered the so-called Dark Ages (ca. 500–1050). Medical and pharmaceutical practice moved into the monasteries and was "transformed into monastic driven system based on religious and superstitious beliefs" (Marriott et al. 2010: 4). The Church questioned the dogma and natural philosophy, so that those who promoted these ideas were treated as heretics and, eventually, persecuted or even slaughtered. Hence, science, including medicine and related studies, had to go underground (Anderson 2005: 32). As a result, the period was characterised by little innovation in the field of medicine and pharmacy. Most of the works of that age are copies of Latin originals that were stored within monasteries. The only and unique non-Latin medical works that preserve traces of classical learning are those written in Anglo-Saxon England (Hunt 1990, Porter 2001)[12].

In the 11th century we can observe a gradual change from the medicine of the Dark Ages to a more thriving field of study. This change was partly influenced by the already flourishing Medical School of Salerno (Italy), parent of great medical schools founded at Montpellier (France), Bologna and Padua (Italy), and later in Oxford and Cambridge (England)[13]. The masters of Salerno "reintroduced theoretical speculation into medical teaching. Aided by contacts with

12 For more on Anglo-Saxon medical texts see section 2.5 in this chapter.

13 For more on universities and schools of medicine see e.g., Bullough (1961, 1962), Siraisi (1990), Norri (1992: 46–53), French (2003: 77–81), Nutton (2011: 153–159), Zebroski (2016: 68–69).

Constantinople, and from 1200 onwards, by Latin translations of some Arabic texts by Constantine the African, they re-established Galenic academic learning, combining commentary on a few texts with philosophical discussion of wider issues (…)" (Porter 2001: 73).

One of the most representative medical works produced at Salerno is *Antidotarium* of Nicolaus Salernitanus (also known as *Antidotarium Nicholai*), which includes from around 110 to 175 recipes (depending on editions), all arranged in alphabetical order. Each prescription starts with the name of a medicine followed by an explanation of the origins of the name and by instructions on how a medicine should be prepared and administered. Moreover, the author of the text systematized the rules of preparing medicaments and introduced a measurement system that allowed physicians and apothecaries to prepare small quantities of pharmaceutical forms. This text, compulsory in a number of universities, became the basis for other pharmaceutical texts produced in medieval Europe (Hunt 1990, Carrillo-Linares 2005, Pocuca — Stupar 2006, Sylwanowicz 2009, Bator — Sylwanowicz 2017a). Another important text of Salerno, *Antidotarium* of Matthaeus Platearius, "based on the work of Dioscorides (…) introduced distillation to European pharmacy and broke away from monastic interpretations by stressing the value of chemistry in medicine" (Anderson 2005: 38).

An important event of that time was the separation of pharmacy from medicine in 1231 as a result of an edict issued by Frederick II of Hohenstaufen (the Emperor of Germany and King of Sicily). This separation was partly influenced by the Arab medicine whose scholars, already in the 9th century, proposed the idea of recognizing pharmacy as distinct from medicine (Hunt 1990: 9). The edict made a clear distinction between physicians and apothecaries, e.g., "(…) physicians and apothecaries could not enter business relationship; the law sought to prevent exploitation of the sick, and there was government supervision of pharmacy. A set dispensatory (list of drugs) had to be used (…). Finally, the druggists (*confectionarii*) and apothecaries (*stationarii*) had to stock certain drugs and keep them no longer than 1 year" (Anderson 2005: 40). These rules, initially executed only in Sicily and southern Italy, became soon a basis for similar legislations across Europe.

The late Middle Ages was a time characterised by a rapid development of medicine towards scholasticism, which treated medicine both as science and craft by combining theory and practice (Pahta — Taavitsainen 2004: 1–2). Besides medical training, doctors, in order to treat their patients correctly, had to be familiar with astrology. Hence, a common feature of many medieval manuscripts is "the zodiac man, depicting the parts of the body and their relationship with the planets and the signs of the zodiac" (Jones 1984: 69). A person born under a certain sign of the zodiac was likely to be influenced by that sign to behave in a certain way. Furthermore, the zodiac man indicated when the moon was in a particular sign, during which period bloodletting or surgical operation would be dangerous for the sick (Norri 1992). Apart from astrological methods, other forms of diagnosis and prognosis were used, for instance, uroscopy (examination of patient's urine), study of physiognomy, observation of blood samples (their colour, consistency, taste, smell and temperature), and diagnosis-prognosis by feeling pulse (recommended by Galen).

The new approach towards medicine was facilitated by translations of Latin and Arabic medical texts into various European vernacular languages. By the 15th century many translated texts circulated through the societies of the Western world, attracting attention of lay readers. This, in turn, resulted in a growing number of non-qualified practitioners who, relying on medical texts, made medical judgements without the aid of medical experts.

Taking into account the discussion above one may conclude that medieval theories of healing played an important part in the development of medicine as science and, as stated by Porter (2001: 81), it was "far from being static, unchanging, or entirely given over to the contemplation of past authorities. It was, in fact, capable of responding effectively to the challenge of disease within its own terms (…)". In addition, towards the end of the period, more and more medical practitioners had the courage to think differently and express their dissatisfaction with ancient traditions employed in medical treatment, which often proved insufficient. This led to a slow rejection of medical practice relying solely on the opinions of authorities (e.g. Hippocratic or Galenic medicine). The outburst of new ideas developed and advanced in the 16th–17th centuries, contributing to the significant changes in practice and theory (Porter 2001: 154, Anderson 2005: 52).

2.3 Medicine in Medieval England[14]

Archaeological excavations reveal that medical practice had been present in the British Isles long before the arrival of the Anglo-Saxons. Medicine was a prestigious occupation for Celts who relied on the experience and wisdom of the Druid priest-healers. According to Griggs (1982: 18–19), certain herbs which were highly valued by the Druids came to be used later by the Anglo-Saxons (Meroney 1945, Norri 1992). Also, during the Roman occupation of Britain, there were

14 This and the following sections are partly based on Sylwanowicz 2014a; the material has been revised and extended.

medical practitioners actively involved in the healing practice. This is mostly evidenced by the instruments and utensils found by archaeologists (Talbot 1967: 9).

The Anglo-Saxons who arrived in the 5th century brought medical concepts rooted in the Teutonic healing practice. For instance, the earliest Germanic practitioners believed in such ideas as (i) sickness as an outcome of elves' actions against people, cf. *ylfa gescotum* 'elfshot, sudden illness'; (ii) the 'worm' as a cause of bodily disorders, cf. *ficwyrm* 'intestinal worm', *toþwyrm* 'worm in tooth' etc.; (iii) the 'flying venom' (cf. *onglyge, ongeflogen*), spreading disease from person to person; and (iv) the belief that number nine was in some way involved in illness and its cure, cf. *The Nine Herb Charm*, the nine herbs to be taken for nine days (Rubin 1974, Norri 1992, Sylwanowicz 2014a: 22).

With the advent of Christianity many pagan ideas were rejected and much emphasis was placed on prayer and God's intervention in healing the sick (Zebroski 2016: 67). Consequently, the Church put more emphasis on the actual words uttered during treatments. Only Christian faith-related words were allowed to be sung, muttered, or spoken, cf. the Old English charm *wið uncuðum swyle* 'for a strange swelling':

(5) Sing on þine læcefinger III Paternoster, and writ ymb þæt sare and cweð: Fuge, diabolus, Christus te sequitur. Quando natus est Christus, fugit dolor. And eft III Paternoster, and III Fuge diabolus. (DOEC, c950, *Anglo-Saxon Charms* (MS Roy 12.D.17), 1–5/17)

As regards a more scholastic approach to medicine, relying on ancient masters such as Galen or Avicenna, it was initially rejected and seen as an intervention against God's will. With time, however, medicine started to be seen as God's gift, and taking responsibility for one's body, being God's creation, began to be a prerogative of every Christian, cf.: "Health obtained through medicine is one of these things that has its origin and existence as a consequence of divine Providence as well as human cooperation" (Amundsen 1996: 135 after Sylwanowicz 2014a: 23).

The changes in the perception of medicine prompted many monks to preserve the medical knowledge of antiquity by copying Latin medical sources that circulated in England as early as the Anglo-Saxon times. Also, Arabic texts attracted the attention of the western medical practitioners, and Latin translations of these texts into English had a considerable influence on the development of medical knowledge (Norri 1992, Sylwanowicz 2014a, Zebroski 2016).

The 14th and 15th centuries, i.e the time when most scientific texts were produced in English, witnessed a rapid advance towards scholasticism and reliance on theoretical foundations derived from antiquity. This is exemplified by frequent references to ancient authorities, found in most medieval English texts, e.g., *Yt is to wyt as seyþ Galien in Metategni…, Ipocras saith that if …, As seiþ Constantinus…, Diascorides seith þat…, Pliniun comaunded…, Aritotil saith…* (Pahta — Taavitsainen 1995, Pahta — Taavitsainen 2004)[15]. Although most late Middle English medical compilations were mere copies of ancient studies, towards the end of this period we can observe a strive for more original concepts.

2.4 Medieval medical practitioners

When a medieval man was looking for medical help, he could turn to a variety of practitioners[16], both learned and non-learned. The first group includes those with a university degree or those who obtained some form of medical instruction at monastic and cathedral schools. The latter group was formed by those who gained medical knowledge through apprenticeship to older and more experienced practitioners or by those who could read and had access to the medical writings (both Latin and English). According to Getz (1998: 5–6), "[they] might have involved themselves in medicine only on occasion, written about it as a part of general knowledge, or healed as a religious duty".

The following sections provide a brief presentation of the most representative groups of those involved in the art of healing in Medieval England[17].

2.4.1 Physicians

The available medieval English sources reflect two sides of the medical world, the learned and the popular. Although no special institution for the training of medical practitioners is known to have existed, the earliest Anglo-Saxon physicians, usually laymen, must have been reasonably well educated since medical documents refer generously to Latin medical texts. Also, a large number of native remedies suggests a relatively high competence of some of Anglo-Saxon physicians,

15 For more on medical authorities in medieval England see, e.g., Matthews (1962), Pahta — Taavitsainen (1995), French (2003), Tavormina (2009).

16 Acording to Getz (1998: 5) "The most distinctive feature of medieval English medicine is indeed the variety of people who practiced it. Unlike other medieval professions that survive today – the ministry, legal and notarial arts, and teaching – medieval medical practice embraced men and women, serfs and free people, Christians and non-Christians, academics and tradespeople, the wealthy and the poor, the educated and those ignorant of formal learning".

17 For a more detailed characteristics of medical practitioners in Medieval England see e.g., Green (1989), Greilsammer (1991), Getz (1998), Nutton (2011: 159–175), Zebroski (2016: 69–71).

often independent practitioners, acting according to their own observations and experience. Their reliance on charm remedies, often containing psalms, litanies or masses to be sung, is good evidence that many physicians were members of monastic communities (Cameron 1993: 19). This implies that monasteries played an important role in the field of medical knowledge. During the Early Middle Ages monastic and cathedral schools sometimes included medicine as one of the subjects, providing students with the basic principles of medical care (Bullough 1966: 36–40). Having access to the medical manuscripts of the monastery, the clergy tended to provide both bodily and spiritual care for the sick inside and outside the cloister walls. However, the emergence of lay leeches suggests that some form of medical learning existed outside monasteries. This practice is estimated to have appeared as early as the pre-Conquest period.

A common Old English noun used with reference to the 'one who heals' was *læce,* with no direct relation to another Old English term *læce* 'a blood-sucking worm' (Carver 1991: 19, Sylwanowicz 2003). The Anglo-Saxon *læce* was a member of *læcecyn* 'a race of physicians or surgeons' and was skilled at *læcecræft*/*læcedom* 'art of healing' and *lacnung* 'medical treatment'. In his practice he often made use of *læceseax* 'surgeon's knife, lancet', *læcewyrt* 'medicinal herb' or *læcesealf* 'salve, ointment', which he often kept in his *læcecyst* 'a medicine chest'. When he was not called to a patient he worked in a *læcehus* 'infirmary, hospital' where he consulted or compiled a *læceboc* 'a book of prescriptions' (TOE, Sylwanowicz 2003).

In the late Middle Ages, universities took over the role of monasteries as centres of medical learning. In Medieval England, the earliest medical faculties were established first in Oxford (late 13th century), and then in Cambridge (late 14th century). As medicine was closely associated with the arts, the student was expected to be skilled in a variety of subjects dealing with the nature of the universe, i.e. natural philosophy (arithmetic, geometry, music, astronomy), rational philosophy (grammar, rhetoric, logic) and moral philosophy (Norri 1992: 47).

Before getting the degree of the Doctor of Medicine, the student was required to complete a 7-year course in arts, after which he could take a course in medicine (about four years), followed by some practical training and delivering lectures (another four years) (Norri 1992: 48). Because typical medical studies took about 17 years, this implies that the medieval physician was a highly learned and versatile man, enjoying a high prestige (French 2003: 1). Thus, the medieval physician was aware of Greek Antiquity and the Muslim world's medical authorities, e.g., Asclepius, Hippocrates, Rhazes or Avicenna. The most influential medical writer was Galen whose "name is perhaps the one which occurs most often on the pages of medieval medical treatises" (Pahta — Taavitsainen 1995: 99). References to Galen and other medical authorities are found in texts belonging to different types of medical writing. For instance, in *Of Phlebotomie*; cf.: "Yt is to wyt as seyþ Galien in Metategni þat if it owth to be done by apofresim, be þe flebotom dippyd in oyle" (Voigts — McVaugh 1984: 39, Pahta — Taavitsainen 1995: 99).

The above described position of a medieval physician is portrayed by Chaucer in the *General Prologue* to the *Canterbury Tales*, cf.:

(6) He knew the cause of everich maladye,
Were it of hoot, or coold, or moyste, or drye,
And where they engendred, and of what humour.
He was a verray, parfit praktisour

(Chaucer, *CT*, G. Prologue (Benson), 419–422)

Chaucer also suggests that "In al this world ne was ther noon hym lik/To speke of phisik and of surgerye" (Chaucer, *CT*, General Prologue (Benson), 412–413).

The changes in the perception of those involved in the art of healing resulted in the modification of the terminology used with reference to medical practitioners. In the 13th and 14th century records we find first attestations of two Romance loanwords, *physician* and *doctor*. The noun *physician* was first used with the meaning 'one who studies natural science or physics (including biology, chemistry and geology)' but soon a *physician* began to be associated with 'someone who practices healing art, both medicine and surgery' (Sylwanowicz 2003), cf. the examples below:

(7) Auh, monie ancren,… þet schulden one lecnen hore soule mid heorte bireousunge and flesshes pinunge, uorwurþeþ **fisiciens** and licomes leches. (OED, a1225 *Ancr. R.* 370)
I am a leche, and with ala good **phesycyen**. (OED, 1484 Caxton *Fables of Æsop* III. ii)

Another term, *doctor*, a derivation from a Latin word meaning 'teacher, instructor', is first recorded as 'one who teaches in some branch of knowledge' (8a). In the course of time the sense developed to 'a knowledgable person' (8b) and finally narrowed down to a more specified meaning 'a knowledgable person practising medicine' (8c), cf.:

(8) a. Saynt Paul, **doctour** of verite. (OED, 1485 Caxton *Chas. Gt.* 1)
b. An introductorie after the statutes of oure **doctours**, in which thou maist lerne a gret part of the generall rewles of theorik in astrologie. (MED, a1450(1391) Chaucer *Astr.* (Benson-Robinson), 117)
c. Maister Gilbert Kymer.. **Doctour** of Medicyns, And Rectour of Medicyns in þe Cite of London. (MED, 1423 *Let.Bk.* in *Bk.Lond.E.* (Gldh LetBk I & K), 108/3)

The introduction of the Romance items overlaps with the formation of medical faculties in the two English leading universities Oxford and Cambridge, which led to the establishment of a hierarchy among medical practitioners. Thus, there occurred a lexical need to make a distinction between a practitioner with academic background (*doctor, physician*) and a *leech* 'a self-trained practitioner'. It is also notable of the English language that, unlike in ancient languages, the terms used with reference to medical practitioners mean both 'healer and teacher'[18].

Women also played an important role in medicine, performing a variety of medical tasks. The Middle Ages offered women three choices in the medical profession: practitioner, midwife and nurse. Because presence of men at birth was often forbidden under death penalty, it was a midwife or a nurse who was allowed to attend child delivery. Most midwives, trained through apprenticeship to older, experienced midwives, generally commanded a good knowledge of herbs. The treatment of wounds, dislocations and fractures was also part of their practice (Norri 1992). Women practitioners were not admitted to universities and, therefore, their knowledge was confined to what they could learn from their male colleagues (Siraisi 1990). There are, however, recorded cases of women "who emerged as learned medical authors who wrote in Latin, drawing on the body of Greco-Islamic source material..." (Siraisi 1990: 27). For instance, Trota, or Trotula, of Salerno, active in the 11th century, is believed to have written a comprehensive treatise on the diseases of women and the care of children. Another, often described, woman practitioner is the Abbess Hildegard of Bingen whose "mystical writings not only make use of medical ideas but also introduce her own idiosyncratic views on female physiology" (Siraisi 1990: 27)[19].

Apart from doctors/physicians who were to "speculate on the cases of illness, erect medical systems, and heal and cure the sick" (Bullough 1966: 109)[20], usually with the help of medications derived from herbs, there was yet another class of practitioners, i.e. surgeons.

2.4.2 Surgeons

Surgery (Gk *cheirourgia* 'working with the hands, the practice of a handcraft or art'; Haubrich 1997: 216) was a profession often seen as a craft. Hence, neither Oxford nor Cambridge offered any surgical training, the only form of learning being experience and apprenticeship.

---

18 The Greeks had the term *iatros* 'healer', whereas the L *medicus* is derived from a verb *medeor* 'to heal' (Charen 1951).

19 For more on medieval women practitioners and patients see, e.g., Power (1922), Hughes (1943), Rowland (1981), Hallaert (1982), Rawcliffe (1995), Kruse (1996, 1999), Green (2000b,c,d, 2001, 2008), Mayer (2008, 2010), Zebroski (2016).

20 For more on medieval English graduates of medical faculty see Bullough (1961: 601–602).

The surgeon was not only expected to perform major operations in which he cut open the patient's body. As Guy de Chauliac states,

(9) [t]he condiciouns þat beþ required in þe Cirurgien beeþ foure/ the ferste is þat// he be a lettred man/ þe secounde þat he be expert or cunnynge/ The þridde þat he be witty or wise/ þe fourþe þat he be wel þewed. It is firste þerfore required þat þe Cirurgien be a lettred man; nogt onliche in þe principles of Cirurgie, but also of phisiqg als wel in theoriqg as in practiqg. (1425, Chauliac, Anatomy (MS Paris angl.25), 25/11–16)

Similar passages are found in most surgical compilations, e.g., in Lanfranc's "Ðe secunde chapitle of þe firste tretis is of þe qualities, maners, and kunnynge of a surgian" (after Fleischhacker 1894: 8). In like manner, John Arderne describes the skills of a surgeon and adds an extensive comment on the key qualities of a surgeon, e.g., piety, charity, modesty, sobriety, courtesy, friendliness to servants and patients, etc. He also emphasises, following the teachings of Avicenna, that "[e]xperience without reason is feble, & so is reson withoute experience fest vnto hym" (after Power 1910: 3).

The Middle Ages can boast of a number of surgical specialists like Guy de Chauliac, Guido Lanfranc, Henri de Mondeville who were the leading medieval authorities that laid foundations for the French Surgery. Of these, Guy de Chauliac was the most influential surgeon of the 14th–15th centuries. He became physician to three popes at Avignon (Clement VI, Innocent VI, and Urban V) and a leading surgeon at the school of Montpellier. As the principal surgical texts of his times, his works were copied and translated into French, English, Italian, Dutch, and even Hebrew (Wallner 1964a: xiii–xviii, Wallner 1971: xiii, Sylwanowicz 2011: 232). Medieval English surgery was represented and influenced by John Arderne who, according to various sources is considered England's first notable surgeon, and by the end of his life obtained the title of Master Surgeon. He is also remembered as the first surgeon to successfully treat Fistula in Ano (a cyst that developed due to long hours spent on a horse) (Power 1910).

Although there was no university faculty specialising in surgery (with the exception of those in Italy), surgeons were expected to have some theoretical background in the field of medicine. According to the sources available, some English surgeons first studied medicine at the universities and afterwards participated in surgical apprenticeship, in order to be admitted to a Guild of Surgeons[21] (Talbot 1967: 120, Norri 1992: 49).

---

21 Since surgery was not taught at medieval universities (except for some universities in Italy), the surgeon's guilds were established to provide practical training (through

Unlike doctors, surgeons were in an unfortunate position, since surgery had a direct causal effect on the health of the patient[22]. Surgeons were often called to perform major operations in which they cut open patients' bodies. Medical doctors, on the other hand, treated most of the patients' illnesses with medications derived from herbs. Most of these herbs did not actually cure the patient, but they also rarely did any harm. Therefore, when a doctor treated a patient, even if the person died, it was difficult to ascribe blame directly to his treatment because most patients got worse over a period of time. However, the surgeon was not as fortunate – the effects of his craft were immediate – the patient either lived or died. Consequently, a large portion of the documentation on surgeons comes from court records concerning malpractice suits (Norri 1992, Sylwanowicz 2014a).

Another group of medical practitioners, who entered the field of surgery, were barbers, untrained artisans who undertook minor surgical operations such as bloodletting or cauterization (Norri 1992). According to Getz (1991: xxviii) barbers were often appointed by London authorities to "prevent the diseased from entering into the city, its prisons, or its baths".

2.4.3 Apothecaries

The study of the history of medicine and pharmacy reveals that originally there was "no real separation of the practice of medicine by the physician from the gatherer of herbs and the preparer of remedies." (Matthews 1962: 1). Thus, anyone involved in the art of healing was expected to be familiar with medical theory on diagnosis and prognosis and, at the same time, be able to prepare certain medicines. However true this statement may be, there are some interesting records that suggest that there were practitioners who were skilled solely in fixing or selling medicines.

In the early Egyptian medical text, *Papyrus Ebers* (ca. 1500 BC), there is a reference to the "Priestly pharmaceutist". In the Bible, we find passages that might be treated as evidence that "the physicians and apothecaries were distinct classes." (Thompson 1929: 14–15)[23].

---

apprenticeship) for the graduates of medical universities who wanted to learn the art of surgery. Thus, a practitioner without a university degree was not admitted to the guild. The apprenticeship varied from five to twelve years. In England, the first surgeon's guild was established in 1368 (cf. Bullough 1966, Beck 1974, Siraisi 1990, Grigsby 1996).

22 For more on surgeons and their instruments see e.g., Wangensteen — Wangensteen (1979), Pouchelle (1990), Hunt (1999), Sylwanowicz (2011).

23 Cf. the Book of Chronicles: "he sought not to the Lord but to the physicians" (2 Chron. 16: 12) and the Book of Nehemiah: "Hananiah, the son of the apothecary," (Neh. 3: 8)

Also in ancient Greece we find distinct classes of those involved in the preparation or trade of drugs. A gatherer of roots and herbs for curative purposes was called *rhizotomist*, whereas the one who sold medicinal substances was referred to as *pharmacopolist*. In the Roman Empire, we find more functions: *seplasiæ* or *seplasiarii* sold medicines, toilet preparations and ointments used in daily hygiene; *pigmentarii* produced dyes and mixed colours, but also prepared and sold medicines ordered by physicians; *pharmacopolists* or *herbalists* sold medicinal plants; *aromatarii* or *confectionarii* fixed and sold aromatic gums and spices; *medicamentarii* gathered roots and plants and sold them to physicians; and *pharmacotribæ* ground spices and made them ready for use. It was also in ancient Rome that the word *apotheca*, from which *apothecary* is derived, was first used with reference to the part of the house where wine, herbs and other products were stored (Thompson 1929: 22–26)[24].

The Arabs are believed to be the first to have established the apothecary's shop (754 AD), and the first to have made the practice of the apothecary distinct from that of a physician (Taylor — Harding 2005). According to Thompson (1929: 82), these apothecaries "were divided into two classes, viz. those who sold simple medicines and non-magistral preparations according to a stated tariff, and the compounders, whose work consisted in scrupulously dispensing the prescriptions of the physicians".

The earliest English "pharmacists" were pepperers and spicers who were mostly involved in a trading activity. Hence the Guild of Pepperers (established in 1180) and the Guild of Spicers (1184). With time, some spicers began to dispense compound medicines and soon began to use the title of apothecary (Anderson 2005: 41, 117, Zebroski 2016: 70). Thus, originally pepperers, spicers and apothecaries were branches of the same group that by the mid-14th century was called the Fraternity of St. Anthony. The only difference was that apothecaries were dealing with drugs for medicinal purposes, whereas the former mostly sold spices and other products employed for domestic purposes (Thompson 1929: 88, Getz 1991: xxix,). In the 15th–16th centuries the group of peppersers, spicers and apothecaries became known as the Grocer's Company, which, apart from pharmaceutical services, had import monopoly on drugs. In this powerful group of merchants, apothecaries formed a small group of individuals who felt overshadowed by other guild members. Therefore, in 1617, by the consent of king James

or the Book of Exodus (30: 35): "And thou shalt make it a perfume, a confection after the art of the apothecary, tempered together, pure and holy." (after Thompson 1929: 15).

24 The shop selling medicines was called *medicina* (Thompson 1929: 26).

I, apothecaries formed their own guild, *The Worshipful Society of the Art and Mystery of the Apothecaries*, which granted them monopoly on selling and preparing medicines (Anderson 2005: 53, 117). Some of the members of the *Society of Apothecaries*, e.g. Sir Theodore Turquet de Mayerne and Gideon de Laune, were regarded as the most influential apothecaries of their times. Both were at the service of the court of James I, and, being allowed to act also as physicians, they left many innovative prescriptions for various ailments (Matthews 1962: 45–53).

Although the earliest status of the apothecary in medical practice and his relationship with physicians is not clearly defined, there are some records which give us a general idea of the position of the compounder of medicines. From Chaucer's *General Prologue* to his *Canterbury Tales* we learn that the doctor "Ful redy hadde he his apotecaries; To sende him drogges and his letuaries" (Chaucer, CT, G. Prologue (Benson), 425–426), which suggests that there must have been some kind of cooperation with and reliance on the skills of apothecaries. However, when there was no apothecary at hand, as Lanfranc notes, a physician had to be ready to make medicines on his own, cf.:

(10) If þou be sent after into a cuntre, þere ben noon apotecarijs, þan if þou canst make þese medicyns þat ben forseid & medicyns þat schulen be seid heraftir, þan þou miȝt fulfille þi purpos. (Fleischhacker, a1400 *LSC1* (MS Ashm 1396), 330/15–18)

There are also documents referring to early English apothecaries that used to be spicers to the kings. For instance, the Pipe Roll of Henry II (1180) states that an apothecary accompanied the king during his journey. The apothecary, known by name and of whom much is known, is Robert de Montpellier, a merchant trader who served Henry III (1207–1272). Although nothing is known of his duties, the records reveal that the king's physician "was required to prepare wines or medicinal substances in the apothecary's presence" (Thompson 1929: 86, Getz 1991: xxix).

Later records, i.e. those from the 16th–17th centuries, give us a better picture of the apothecary and his duties. In the mid-16th century *Government of Health* by William Bullein[25] we find a thorough description of the apothecary, cf.:

(11) He must fyrst serve God, forsee the end, be clenly, pity the poor. Must not be suborned for money to hurt mankynde. (…) His garden must be at hand with plenty of herbs, seeds and roots. To sow and gather, preserve and kepe them in due tyme. To read Dioscorides, to know the nature of plants and herbes. To invent medicines, to choose colours, taste, odour, figure, etc. (…) That he neither increase nor diminish the Phisician's bill and kepe it for his discharge. (…) That he delyte to reede

25 William Bullein was a 16th century physician, botanist and rector of Balxhall, Suffolk.

> Nicholas Myrepsus, Valerius Cordus, Johannes Placaton, the Lubik, etc. That he do remember that his office is only to be ye physician's cooke. That he use true measure and weight (…). (after Thompson 1929: 162–163)

As the description above reveals, an apothecary was required to have an extensive knowledge about the qualities and ways of preservation of the herbs, spices and other substances used in fixing medicines. In addition, he was expected to be familiar with the works of various medical authorities and be able to invent his own medicines. Last, but not least an apothecary should be modest and trustworthy, and remember that his primary duty was to be the "physician's cooke" (Thompson 1929: 162–163).

Interestingly, there is a manuscript entitled *A Booke of plaisters, spasmadraps, ointments, pulthes, etc. devysed by the King's Majestie, Dr. Butts, Dr. Chambre, Dr. Cromer and Dr. Augustin,* which provides evidence that Henry VIII had special interest in the work of an apothecary. Many of the prescriptions included in the text, especially those applied externally, were probably composed by the king himself who suffered from various ailments of the legs. Thus, we find the following prescriptions: *The King's Majestie's Own Plaster, A plaster devysed by the King's Majestie to resolve and cease payne…, A Plaster of the King's to heale and drye made at St. James*, etc. (Thompson 1929: 168–173).

2.5 Medieval English medical sources

Anyone involved in the medical use or making of medicines required a solid knowledge about them. This knowledge was disseminated through the word of mouth or, most often, through the manuscripts. Before the introduction of printing these texts required from a monk copying by hand, which often took years, if not decades. Hence, originally, medical know-how was reserved to only a few. It was the invention of printing that gave access to a large number of medical sources and spread the knowledge of the art of healing to a wider audience. What follows is a brief presentation of the chief medical works produced in Medieval England.

According to Cameron (1993), the oldest surviving English medical text, dated back to about 850–900, is the so-called *Omont* fragment. It is a single leaf containing on the recto page names of several remedies dealing with the ailments of the foot, leg, thigh, and with paralysis. The verso page contains practice alphabets and designs.

A larger and more representative collection of texts dates back to the 10th century. They were compiled and edited by Oswald Cockayne in the Rolls Series between 1864 and 1866, as *Leechdoms, Wortcunning and Starcraft of Early England.*

The collection is divided into three books, Book I and Book II (Bald's *Leechbook*) and Book III (*Leechbook* III). The first two books deal with external (Book I) and internal disorders (Book II), and they rely heavily on classical sources. The third book (*Leechbook* III), on the other hand, deals entirely with native medicine. Cockayne's work includes also a collection of medical prescriptions referred to as *Lacnunga*. The manuscript deals mostly with folk medicine compiled randomly by non-medical scribes. It abounds in prescriptions and remedies of magical character (Cameron 1993).

Another group of Old English texts constitute translations of the following Latin works: *Herbarium of Apulei*, a description of herbs and plants, and *Peri Didaxeon*, a collection of non-Salernitan medical treatises originally known as the *Practica Petrocelli Salernitani* (or *Petrocellus* in short) (Voigts 1979, Cameron 1993).

The body of Middle English medical writings is much more extensive. According to Singer (1919), apart from a large number of medical compilations in Latin or Greek (altogether about 7000), there were at least 1032 Middle English medical writings produced in the 13th–15th centuries (cf. also Robbins 1970: 393).

A large number of these texts prompted many linguists to categorise them in a number of ways. Robbins (1970) suggested to divide the texts on the basis of their content, namely: diagnosis, prognosis, and treatment. The division, however, has certain drawbacks. First of all, a particular text often includes material representing all the three areas mentioned by Robbins, while many academic treatises first define sickness, and then discuss its causes, symptoms, prognosis and cure (Norri 1992: 34).

The next division of texts is that of Voigts (1982) and Voigts — McVaugh (1984), who proposed to break down Middle English medical texts according to their origin (e.g. translations of classical works and collections produced in English), and intended audience (learned and non-learned). This division was picked up by the editors of MEMT who classified the Middle English corpus into three main categories: (i) surgical texts, (ii) specialised treatises, and (iii) remedies and *materia medica* (Taavitsainen — Pahta — Mäkinen 2005). The first two collections include texts representing the learned tradition of writing. These texts, written and/or translated by university-trained physicians, were mostly compilations referring to ancient Latin, Arabic or contemporary medieval medical works. Texts in these collections were mostly theoretical writings dealing with a specific field of specialisation or medical problems, e.g. instructions for surgical practitioners, treatises on the sicknesses of women, discussions of various treatments, e.g., for fistula, gout, ulcers, excessive bleeding, etc. The third collection of medical writings consists mostly of remedies, i.e. books for consultation which represent the earliest phase of vernacular medicine, established already in Old English (cf. Taavitsainen 2001, Sylwanowicz 2014a, 2016). They belong to the lower, non-learned layer of medical practice, the largest part of these collections constituting recipes, i.e. instructions on how to fix medical preparations or how to deal with a medical problem. This classification suggests a clear-cut division into the intended audience: surgical and specialised texts written for the learned audiences, and remedy book collections for the less learned. However, the fact that surgical and specialised texts were translations from classical languages suggests that they were not necessarily intended solely for educated audiences (cf. also Alonso Almeida — Carroll 2004). Similarly, in the group of remedy books, often described as less dependent on foreign models, there are collections which rely heavily on Latin originals written by university-trained practitioners (e.g. a collection of recipes labelled as *Antidotarium Nicholai*).

Alonso Almeida — Carroll (2004) proposed yet another classification of medical texts, i.e. theory-only books (booklets, individual texts dealing with anatomy, surgery, etc.), practice-only books (recipe books and prescriptions) and theory-practice books including texts that are "in an intermediate position between learned texts and popular remedy books" (Alonso Almeida — Carroll 2004: 32). This division is also not free of shortcomings. For instance, in which category should one include the surgical works of Lanfranc or Arderne, which, apart from theoretical treatises on various medical problems, include also instructions on how to prepare medicaments (recipes). Surely, they cannot be included in the third category proposed by the authors, as they are examples of highly technical texts directed at experienced surgeons rather than amateur healers.

The present study follows the taxonomical model proposed by the editors of MEMT. This allows one to observe differences in the choice of the terminology (here: names of medical preparations) from medieval medical compilations that represented different writing traditions (remedy books, surgical texts and specialised treatises). A preliminary investigation of these texts has revealed that the use or avoidance of specialised terminology might have been determined by the text's intended audience. For instance, in the recipe collections included in the category remedy books, there is a relatively lower number of names of medicaments than in specialised texts. This is often explained by the fact that the users of these collections were not always familiar with medical nomenclature. Hence, in these writings the compilers tended to state the purpose of the recipe, specifying the medical problem to be cured, rather than provide the name of the preparation.

2.6 Medieval English recipes[26]

Since the aim of this work is a thorough study of the names of medicaments, what follows is a brief characteristics of Middle English recipe collections, i.e. instructions on how to prepare a medicine.

English medieval medical recipes are mostly translations or adaptations from Latin and Anglo-Norman originals which follow the traditions of scientific writing established by Latin medical writers. Thus, in the earliest English medical texts we can find English recipes in company with Latin/Anglo-Norman samples. The predominantly English compilations became widespread in the second half of the 15th century, which was partly facilitated by the introduction of the printing press in 1476.

Medical recipes are mostly found in remedy books, i.e. texts representing the oldest tradition of medical writing. As Taavitsainen (2001: 85–86) observes, these recipes "are a well-defined procedural genre with a clear writing purpose" and their text type features show "a high degree of standardization". Their content is fairly uniform: they usually consist of a title (12a) or a statement of their purpose (12b), followed by a list of ingredients, instructions on how to prepare a medicament, administration of a preparation, justification of use and additional information (Taavitsainen 2001: 86, Mäkinen 2004: 146)[27].

(12) a. **ADRIANUM**. Yt ys cleped of Adryan, Emperor of Rome, þe wyche yt compownde. Yt ys goode properlyche to alle [\f. 3r\] euel of þe hed of coldnes, and to greuance of þe eyȝen, and to derkenes of hem, and to the mygrayne. Take opium theobaicum, III dragmes; cassia lignea, henebane sed, of eyþer [{II{] dragmes II scripules and half; ewforbe, whyte peper, of eche II dragmes and VI corne wyght and þe þridde parte of a corne of whete; (...) Be yt [\f. 3v\] ȝeue wyþ hote weyne in þe wyche sauge hathe be ysode ynne in þe maner of an auellane. Be yt ȝefe to hem þat haueþe þe feuere quarteyne wyþ decoction of gencyan or wylde rewe, byfore the howre of acces. Be yt ȝef alsoo to þe pacyent þat bygynneþ to haue the ston wyþ wyn in þe wyche gromyle or saxifrage haþe be sode ynne. (MEMT, 15th c. *AntN* (MS Ferguson 147), f. 2v)

b. **An electuarie þat restoriþ a man-is mynde and comforteþ his brayn and / al his body**: Take of canel, roses, violet, ginger, cardamomum, of eueriche, oz. ii; of dragagantum, antos, bawme þat ia an herbe, maioran, þe rynde of myrtille,

26 This section is partly based on Bator—Sylwanowicz (2017b).

27 For more on the structure of Middle English recipes see, e.g., Stannard (1982), Hunt (1990), Görlach (1992), Taavitsainen (2001), Mäkinen (2004, 2006), Carroll (1999, 2004), Jones (1998a), Alonso Almeida (1998, 1999, 2013), Bator—Sylwanowicz (2017b), Cruz-Cabanillas (2017).

ciperi, liquoris, siler, of eueriche, oz. ii; of squinantum, spike, clowes, quibibis, folii, galange, auence, borage, sene, bean, spodie, coral, mastike, macropipir, storax, brent silke, of eueriche, oz. ½ & sc. i; of sirep of roses, quantum sufficit. (Getz, a1475 *GA* (MS Wel 537), 20/6–14)

Recipes are not confined to remedy books alone, being also found in scientific texts, where they form an integral part of longer treatises, hence, their structure is often not that regular as in remedy books. The difference in content and the internal structure of recipes allows one to distinguish at least three types of recipes, i.e. *antidotaria, receptaria* and *experimenta* (cf. Hunt 1990, Mäkinen 2004).

Antidotaria recipes are often called full recipes (see 12a above) as they contain all the elements characteristic of the structure of a recipe text, i.e. name/title, list of ingredients and their measures, as well as their preparation and application (Hunt 1990: 8). The remedies included in *antidotaria* are of a learned character, i.e. no folk element is included, and the weights and measures are usually precise and detailed (Hunt 1990, Mäkinen 2004).

The *receptaria*, unlike *antidotaria*, are much shorter texts, found in medical rather than strictly pharmaceutical texts. They are usually part of longer medical treatises and arranged according to their purpose (see 12b above). Thus, most *receptaria* are recognized by the following introductory lines: *A (good, special) medicine for…*, *Another (medicine) for…*, followed by the name of the sickness or a statement of purpose (Getz 1991, Mäkinen 2004). These short recipes often incorporate folk medicine and are characterized by the use of less precise measure terms, e.g., *a little, a quantity of*, though specified terms are also found, but less frequently (cf. also Bator — Sylwanowicz 2017a).

The last category of recipes, *experimenta*, are not found in medical or pharmaceutical compilations as they are short passages, being passed down by word of mouth, "jotted down after hearing them from a colleague or an acquaintance who had proved the efficacy of the recipe in practice." (Mäkinen 2004: 147).

2.7 Products of pharmacy

In medieval medical practice the therapeutic use of substances depended largely on the humoral medicine, which classified medicines according to what humours they eliminated. Hence, the division into cold, hot, dry and moist medicines (Getz 1991, Anderson 2005, Sylwanowicz 2009). Accordingly, all diseases were identified by the same properties and it was advised to treat them by medicines with opposite properties. For instance, in an English version of *Gilbertus Anglicus* (a 15th century rendering of a 12th century Latin compilation), a pain in eyes (being a hot disease) is treated with cold medicines (Getz 1991, Sylwanowicz 2009: 350), cf.:

(13) Special medicyns for ache of yȝen þat comeþ hete, as of blode þat is hote and moyst, or of coler þat is hote and drye, þei muste be colde forto be, mytigatiues, þat is to sey, to aswage þe violence of þe ache. And þey must be colde to be repercussyues, þat is to sey, to smyten aȝen fro þe yȝe þe humour þat is cause of þe ache. (Getz, a1475 *GA* (MS Wel 537), 36/5–11)

Treating illnesses with the substances of opposite properties was not a general rule and we find sources proposing that some ailments should be treated with medicines of the same quality, i.e. cold disease with a cold remedy, etc. (Sylwanowicz 2009: 350), cf.:

(14) But neuertheles otherwhiles syknes ben iheled with medicynes that ben accordyng with hem and nat with contrarie thynges (…). For yf a mannys hed be right hote and he put it in to cold watir outher in to snow it shal be moche more hottir than it was before. And the cause is for the colde stoppeth the poores and closeth the hete withynforth in lesse place than it was before and euery thyng is of grettir myght whan it is to gedir than it is departed abrood. (MEMT, 15th c. *ThP* (MS Sln 3489), f. 32r)

In her discussion of the Middle English version of *Gilbertus Anglicus*, Getz notices that medicines were recognised as general, all-purpose remedies, and as specifics that were used to treat particular illnesses. To support her findings, Getz (1991: xl) provides the following fragment: "a profitable salt and a thing that purges all humors in a person's head, and it is good for aching of the joints, and for the gout, and for the dropsy". This quotation is followed by fragments describing similar properties of sugars (of borage, of roses or of violets). As for specifics (ointments, powders, oils, waters, plasters, syrups, pills, etc.), we can find numerous references in both Middle and Early Modern English medical texts. These substances, can be grouped according to the same classification that is used today, i.e. liquids, semi-solids and solids[28].

Medicines were also classified into those applied internally or externally, e.g.:

(15) For thyes maner of diseasys may not be curid oonly by medycyns, neyther **ynward or outwarde** nor princypally, but by thys craft that ys callyd "ars acuaria," that ys to saye the craft of nedyl. (MEMT, 1474–1499 *BG* (MS Hunter V.8.6), 54)
(…) put no medycyne nor **withyn nor wythoute,** ffor þis infi rmytee may not be curyd wyth laxatyvs nor wyth pouders nor wyth coleryes nor wyth electuaryes nor wyth cauteryes (…). (MEMT, 1474–1499 *BG* (MS Hunter V.8.6), 62–63)

28 For a more detailed discussion on the division into dosage forms see chapter four.

or into simple and compound. The difference between these two is explained in the following passage:

(16) But þou muste vndirstonde **þat of þes medicyns, sum ben simple and sum ben componed.** Simple medicyns ben, as of oon herbe by himsilf, or of oon watir þat is y-made of oon herbe, or of hony, or of oyle de olif, or of oon gumme, or of oon spicery by him-silf. **Componed medicens ben made of two** þingis, or þre, or of meny þingis y-medlid togederis. (Getz, a1475 *GA* (MS Wel 537), 37/9–15)

Simple medicines involved one ingredient, e.g., one herb with medicinal properties. This herb was applied either in a powdered form or as the only ingredient of some liquid medicine (water or oil). Therefore, simple medicines are usually found in herbals or in other compilations describing, among others, the healing properties of herbs, spices or minerals (e.g. stones). Compound medicines, as the name suggests, are usually compositions of two or more herbs, oils, waters, or other ingredients. The earliest practitioners preferred simples as it was in accordance with the Galenic claim that simples were "God-given cures" and any compounding was a blasphemy as it was showing that God's creation was imperfect and insufficient (cf. Wear 2000: 96).

Another classification of remedies divides them according to their properties, i.e. medicines that are strong, sharp, easy, bitter, cleaning, cooling, light, hard, great, cf.:

(17) **medicynes** bene **bitter** or **sharp** or sich other (Power, 1425 *AFS* (MS Sln 6), 7/6–7)
many propertes of **oyntmenttes** in store with in hym þat ys to say (…) a **clensynge onyment** a **kelynge onyment** and an **hetynge onyment.** (MEMT, 1500 *BS* (MS Hrl 1736), f. 7r)
And it shal be helid by **corrosyues, confortatiues, repercussiues, mytigatiues, and strictories,** and blood-lettinggis, like as obtalmie is y-helid. (Getz, a1475 *GA* (MS Wel 537), 51/10–12)

The examples reveal that early medical practitioners were well aware of various properties of the substances they used and, despite variation in the classification of these items, they were fairly consistent in their use. Additionally, one can conclude that the earliest classifications of medicines laid foundations for the modern typology of pharmaceuticals.

Chapter three: General terms denoting medical preparations

3.1 Introduction: selection and classification

The present chapter centres on Middle English nouns referring to 'any substance or preparation used in the treatment of disease' (OED, *medicine* n.[1]) in general, i.e. lexemes that could be used as potential primary terms for the lexical category 'medical preparations'. The list does not include nouns that denote dosage forms, i.e. lexemes that denote physical characteristics (solid, semi-solid or liquid) of a given medicament, e.g., *ointment, pill, syrup*, or names of specifics, i.e. lexemes that denote preparations aimed to treat particular ailment and/or part of the body, e.g., *apostolicon, diamoron, gargarisma, hiera pigra*, etc.

A difficulty one encounters here is that of delimitation, i.e. which items could be included as potential members of the field. A line had to be drawn somewhere to eliminate items that could not be treated as representative. Chapter three contains a review of the principles of the selection of relevant nouns, discusses their etymology, use and distribution in the material gathered for this study.

As a starting point, the *Dictionary of Medical Vocabulary in English, 1375–1550* (DMVE), *Middle English Dictionary* (MED), *Oxford English Dictionary* (OED), and the *Historical Thesaurus of English* (HTE) were searched. However, dictionary definitions of selected nouns vary, which makes it difficult to decide on the spot whether an item could be treated as a general term denoting 'a medical preparation'. Therefore, it was necessary to read the Middle English medical texts thoroughly in order to find text samples that would eliminate any doubts concerning meanings of the nouns. Also, it seemed possible that medical writings might contain nouns different from those listed in the dictionaries.

According to HTE, the earliest English lexemes (till 1550) used with reference to 'a medical preparation' were: *caulic, (ge)lacnung, lybb,* and *pigment*. Of these, according to MED, only *(ge)lacnung* and *pigment* were recorded in Middle English writings. The first, in the form *lechnunge* (also *lacnunge, lacninge*), was found to denote healing or spiritual remedy, whereas the latter was used with the sense 'spice; remedy containing spices' or 'a red dye' (cf. MED, *lechnunge* ger., and *pigment* n.). Later examples listed by HTE include *dia*[29], *drug, medicament,*

29 According to MED the form *dia* is found with the sense 'a pharmaceutical preparation, a medicament'. The form is derived from the Latin prefix *dia-* 'made of' which is found

medicinal, medicine, pharmacy, receipt, treacle. DMVE, MED and OED reveal that the list seems incomplete and the nouns *antidote, boot, confection, cure, help, leechcraft, leechdom, physic, remedy, spice, tiriac* are suggested as possible Middle English general referents to 'a medical preparation'. A thorough reading of the medical material collected for the present work supplies us with additional two nouns: *helping* and *health*.

The preliminary investigation yielded 21 Middle English nouns as possible general referents to a 'a medical preparation, medicament', cf.:

> *antidote, boot, confection, cure, dia, drug, help, helping, health, leechcraft, leechdom, medicament, medicinal, medicine, pharmacy, physic, receipt, remedy, spice, tiriac, treacle.*

The analysis of the medical material has shown that some of the nouns suggested by dictionaries cannot be considered as representative examples of the category 'general terms denoting medicines'. These nouns can be divided into the following groups: (a) nouns (*dia, drug, leechdom, medicament*) that have not been found in the examined medical texts at all, (b) nouns (*cure, leechcraft, physic, medicinal*) that have been documented in medical texts with the sense other than 'a medical preparation', and (c) nouns (*health, pharmacy, treacle*) recorded as referents to medicinal substances of specific character. What follows is a brief discussion of these terms.

Dia, drug, leechdom and *medicament* are the only nouns from the list that have not been recorded in the medical writings collected for the present study. This, however, does not imply that a medieval physician or anyone involved in the healing practice was unfamiliar with these nouns. On the contrary, as the quotations from MED and OED reveal, the nouns might have been commonly known everyday words used with reference to any 'medical preparation', cf.:

(18) And dryuen awey deth with **dyas** and **dragges**. (OED, 1377 Langl. *P.Pl.* B. xx. 173)
Dragge nor **dya** was noon in Bury toun.
(MED, c1460 (?c1435) *Lydg. Let.Glo.* (MS Hrl 2255) 12)
Apothecaries To sende hym **drogges** (OED, c1386 Chaucer Prol. 428)
Raphaæl bitacneþþ uss..Drihhtiness hallȝhe **læchedom** & sawless eȝhesallfe..he wollde himm senndenn Wiþþ heofennlike **læchedom** To læchenn Tobess eȝhne. (MED,?c1200 *Orm. (Jun 1)* 1851, 1855)
Other take Her scions fild with this **medicament** [theriac].
(MED,?1440 *Palladius* (MS DukeH d.2) 3.1110)

---

in the names of medical preparations (MED *dia*, n. and *dia*-, pref.). Its function was to indicate the main ingredient (cf. also chapter 5, section 5.2.1).

Thus, it can be assumed that the nouns were part of a non-specialised register. But it is surprising to learn that *leechdom*, a very frequent noun found already in Old English[30] medical works with at least two medical senses, i.e. 'a prescribed medicine, remedy' (19a) or 'a medical prescription' (19b), is not recorded in Middle English medical corpora.

(19) a. **Læcedomas** gif men yrne blod of nebbe, eft blodsetena ge onto bindanne ge on eare to donne ge horse ge men. (DOEC, Cockayne, *Bald's Leechbook*, II, 2–16)
b. **Læcedomas** wiþ sarum weolorum. (DOEC, Cockayne, *Bald's Leechbook*, II, 18–156)

One of the possible explanations for no records of *leechdom* in Middle English medical writings is suggested by the editors of MED who indicate that in the 13th century the noun started to be replaced by another Old English noun, *leechcraft*. Originally, this term was used with the following senses: 'art of healing/medical science' (20a), 'remedy/medicine' (20b) and/or 'prescription' (20c), cf.:

(20) a. Witodlice þær wæs sum munuc, þam wæs namalustus, se wæs gelæred on **læcecræfte**, (…). (DOEC, Hecht, *Gregory the Great, Dialogues*, 179–259)
b. Genim geoluwne stan salt stan pipor weh onwæge drif þurh clað do ealra gelice micel do eal togædere drif eft þurh linene clað. Þis is afandan **læcecræft**. (DOEC, Cockayne, *Recipes*, I, 374–378)
c. Þis ys þe **læcecræft**: Sule hym supan gebræddan hrere ægeran and hunig to and do hym bryð of meolce gemaced, and syle hym ceruillan etan and fæt flæsc, þæt beo wel gesoden, etan, and he byd sona hal. (DOEC, L[ouml]weneck, *Peri Didaxeon*, 3–53)

Despite the variety of medical senses, the noun, compared with *leechdom*, was less frequently used in Old English medical writings, with only 7 records.

In the Middle English period, as MED suggests, *leechcraft* retained its original senses and unlike *leechdom*, the noun was still used in medical manuals. However, as the analysis of the material gathered for the present study has revealed, the noun has been found only in the sense 'art of medicine; remedy', cf.:

(21) Þese.vj. þingis (…) techiþ a man speculatijf of **leche craft**. (Fleischhacker, a1400 *LSC1* (MS Ashm 1396), 17/10)
(…) shulde renne to medecyne.i. lechecrafte and shulde be made leches. (Wallner, 1425 *GCA1* (MS NY 12), 26/10–11)

The noun *cure* (derived from OF *cure* and L *cura* 'care'), whose general reference to a medical substance is also questionable, entered English in the first half of

30 A thorough reading of Old English texts has yielded at least 236 records of the noun *leechdom*.

the 14th century and was used with a variety of senses relating to the act of care, attention or concern. With time, i.e. around 1380 (cf. MED, *cure* n.[1]), the noun started to be used in a medical context in the sense of 'medical/surgical treatment or case' and this sense is recorded in the texts studied, cf.:

(22) Þis womman was vndir þe **cure** of a ȝong man þat was my scoler. (Fleischhacker, a1400 *LSC1* (MS Ashm 1396), 221/2–3)
At last I..did my **cure** to hym. (Power, 1425 *AFS* (MS Sln 6), 1/22–23)

Although MED suggests that the noun denoted also 'a medical preparation' no such record has been found in the medical manuals examined for the present work.

Similarly, *physic* (from OF *fisique* 'natural science, art of healing' and L *physica* 'study of nature') is not documented in the examined material in the sense 'a medical preparation', though MED states the opposite. However, the quotations given by the dictionary come from non-medical writings, cf.:

(23) He..nom wiþ him spicerie þat to **fysike** drou. (MED, c1325 (c1300) *Glo.Chron.A* (MS Clg A.11) 3162)
The Frere with his **phisik** þis folke hath enchaunted, And plastred hem so esyly þei drede no synne. (MED, c1400(c1378) *PPl.B* (MS LdMisc 581) 20.376)

In the medical material analysed for this study the records of *physic* (about 15 hits) denote 'medical science', cf.:

(24) In þe morning bifore þu [{go{]st furth, vse certeine electuaryis aftir þe councell of men experte in **phisike**. (MEMT, 1500 *RS* (Rwl C.83), 5)
(…) it is nessessarie a surgian to knowe **phisik**, & oþer dyuers science, as I haue told tofore in þe book. (Fleischhacker, a1400 *LSC1* (MS Ashm 1396), 18/9–10)

Medicinal is another term whose reference to medical preparations in medieval context is dubious. The earliest OED quotation for *medicinal* with the sense 'medical preparation' is dated back to 1667, e.g., "In Medicinals we have now and then..inquired after some rarities." (OED, H. Oldenburg in *Philos. Trans.* (Royal Soc.) 2 410). Other sources, i.e. MED and medical texts collected for the present work, reveal that in the Middle English writings the term is recorded only as an adjective describing medical means, theory or science, cf.:

(25) Þe **medicynal** instrumentis ben dietis. pociouns. bloodles. oynementis. emplastris & poudris. (Wallner, 1425 *GCM* (MS Cai 336/725), 9/4–5)
Y wyl delyure to þe techinge **Medicynal** and conseilys þat shal suffyce þe in kepyng of hele. (MED, a1500(?a1425) *Lambeth SSecr.* (MS Lamb 501), 66/13)
Therfore he þat wole knowe what siurgie is, he moot vndirstonde, þat it is a **medicinal** science, which techiþ us to worche wiþ handis in mannes bodi. (Fleischhacker, a1400 *LSC1* (MS Ashm 1396), 7/15)

The next group of nouns, *health*, *pharmacy*, *tiriac* and *treacle*, classified according to HTE as general terms for 'a medical preparation', are documented in the examined material with reference to 'medicaments of specific character'.

According to DMVE, MED and OED, *health* (from OE *hælþ*) was not recorded in Middle English writings as a simple term denoting 'a medical preparation'. This is supported by a careful reading of the medical texts where the noun is used in phrases rendering the following Latin names for pharmaceuticals: (i) L *universalibus antydotis* 'a medical preparation for treating disorders of various parts of body', (ii) L *antidotis particularibus* 'a medical preparation for treating disorders in particular body part, e.g. head, face, neck', (iii) L *antidotis localibus* 'a medical preparation applied locally, e.g. ointment'; cf. DMVE (*health* n.) and the following quotation:

(26) Here bygynneþ the .7. tretys þat is saide an Antidotarie (…) [;] the firste is of **vnyuersal helþes** or helpes. The secounde schal be of **particuler helþes** (…) / The .6. chapitle is of **stedefast helþes** of woundes & of bocches (…). (Wallner, *GCA2* (MS Paris angl. 25), 51/8–10, 30)

In addition, the noun is underrepresented in the medical material, as it has been recorded only 4 times in a single surgical text (one of the 15th century English translations of Guy de Chauliac's treatise on *Anatomy*)[31].

The term *pharmacy* (from OF *farmacie* 'purgative', L *pharmacia* 'use of medicines'), following DMVE and MED, also denoted some specifics, i.e. 'medicines that purged the body of an excess of any humour except blood', cf.:

(27) Fleobotomye or **farmacie** solueþ or leseþ aking of yen. (MED,?a1425 **Chauliac(1)* (NY 12) 39a/a)
Superflue humourez al, outake blode, bene to be purged by **farmacie**. (MED,?a1425 **Chauliac(1)* (NY 12) 158b/a)
Þe firste [probleme] is which ben purge wiþ medcyn laxatif.s. **farmacia**. (DMVE, a1425 **Chauliac(2)* (Jes-C Q.G.23) 360 rb)

---

31 Two English versions of Guy de Chauliac's treatise on Anatomy have been analysed: MS N.Y. (preserved in the Library of the New York Academy of Medicine) and MS A. (kept in the National Library in Paris). The translators of these two versions differed significantly in their choice of the terms. MS N.Y. is generally characterised by the use of words of Latin or French origin, while in MS A. we can observe a tendency to use vernacular items. For instance, where MS N.Y. has *antidoteȝ*, the translator of MS A. uses the term *helthe*, e.g., *antidoteȝ or helpyngeȝ* (N.Y.) vs. *helþes or helpes* (A.), *antidoteȝ locales* (N.Y.) vs. *stedefast helþes* (A.). In the present work MS N.Y. is referred to as GCA1, and MS A. as GCA2. For more on the differences between MS N.Y. and MS A. see, for instance, Wallner (1964b) and Sylwanowicz (2009, 2011).

The quotations above suggest also that *pharmacy*, if used in a medical text, was restricted to surgical compilations. This assumption is supported by a thorough reading of the medical corpora gathered for the present study. The noun is recorded only in surgical writings (54 hits), whose compilers explain that *pharmacy* is a laxative medicine, cf.:

(28) (…) as **farmacye or laxing** nedeþ dyete right so nedeþ cirurgie dyete & farmacie. (Wallner, 1425 *GCA2* (MS Paris angl. 25), 27/3–4)
Þe bodi war first mundified with **farmacie.i. medicyne laxatiue**. (Power, 1425 *AFS* (MS Sln 6),68/22–23)
A walkynge Vleus ys y-helyde with flebotomye & **ffarmasye þat is laxatyfes** purgynge (…). (Fleischhacker, a1450 *LSC2* (MS Add 12056), 83/38–39)

Similarly, *tiriac* (from L *theriaca* 'antidote for poisonous wild animals') and *treacle* (from OF *triacle* 'antidote, cure for snake-bite') should not be recognised as general terms for medicines. These terms denoted a compound medicine, including multiple ingredients, that was one of the most popular and valuable medieval medicaments that had been known since the ancient times (Nockels-Fabbri 2007: 248–252). Originally, these nouns denoted 'an antidote for poison or venom; a medicament for drawing out or neutralizing the poison engendered by infection, suppuration, etc.;' (MED, *tiriake* n. and *triacle* n.), cf.:

(29) Lete hym holde in his mouþe þese pelotis. Recipe **tiriace** [L: tyriace (16va)], rubee trociscate [etc.]. (DMVE, c1425 **BernLiliyum* (MS Ashm 1505), 149r)
Hit is nedeful..to drinke triacle wiþ hote wyne and to smere þerwith þe sore place, for if þe **triacle** is ipreued and hit be a verray antrax, þe triacle schal drawe out þe matiere þat is drye & venemous. (MED, a1398 *Trev.Barth.* (MS Add 27944), 419/14–16)
This **triacle** is good for men þat ben y-poisened or biten of venemous bestis or wormes, or of woode ho[u]nde. (Getz, a1475 *GA* (MS Wel 537), 152/6–8)

With time, the preparation started to be recognised as a universal remedy against various sicknesses or morbid conditions, e.g. fevers, problems with the liver, indigestion, stones in kidneys, strangury, palsy or even the plague[32] (30a). In places, this medicament is listed as one of the ingredients of other medicinal substances (30b), cf.:

(30) a. And so þou mai do þerof if a mannes liuer is distemperid with heet and in dissinterie also. And if al þis helpiþ him not, ȝyue him gode **triacle**, for þat staunchiþ eueri flux. (Getz, a1475 *GA* (MS Wel 537), 189/15–18)

---

32 *Treacle* was also "believed to possess virtually magical powers" (Nockels–Fabri 2007: 252).

b. On suppositorie is this: Take **triacle** diatesseron +Q sem. and of cocle floure as moche (...) then make hit vp with cotton & therof make a suppositorie as gret as thy litell fynger and putte in her prevy membre. (Rowland, 1450 *SW2* (MS Sln 2463), 68/14–18)

Although *tiriac* and *treacle* are fairly well represented in medical writings (34 hits) there is no evidence that might allow one to include them in the list of potential members of general names for medicines.

Taking into account the discussion above, the final selection of potential general terms denoting 'a medical preparation' yielded 3 terms of Old English heritage (*boot*, *help*, *helping*) and 6 Middle English adoptions of Romance terms (*antidote*, *confection*, *medicine*, *receipt*, *remedy* and *spice*). All these nouns are recorded in the medical writings examined for the present study with the sense 'a medical preparation'. Table 1 shows the distribution of these terms in the analysed material.

Tab. 1: The number of the occurrences (absolute frequencies) of general terms for 'a medical preparation' in the analysed material

Old English heritage	Number of occurrences	Romance adoptions in Middle English	Number of occurrences
help	6	**medicine**	1047
helping	3	**confection**	49
boot	1	**antidote**	13
		remedy	7
		receipt	6
		spice	2

3.2 Old English heritage

Boot, *help* and *helping* are the nouns that had been recorded with a medical meaning already in the Old English texts. They, however, were not restricted to the medical context and were common every-day words used with a variety of senses not associated with the medical realm. Therefore, if found in Middle English medical manuals it is not always easy to deduce their actual reference. This might also explain their peripheral use in the analysed texts (cf. Table 1).

One of the earliest records suggests that *boot* was originally used with two senses: 'a remedy' or 'a medicine', which is documented by the following quotations from MED and OED:

(31) Þe eow eagena leoht, fram blindnesse **bote** gefremede. (OED, a1000 Cynewulf *Elene* 299)
Min heoueneliche leche þet makedest us of þi seolf se mihti medicine..hit beo mi lechunge, hit beo mi **bote**. (MED, a1250 *Orison Lord* (MS Lamb 487), 187)

In Middle English medical writings, the word is recorded only once alongside the noun *remedy* (see 32 below). Taking into account the fact that even today *remedy* is often understood either as a treatment or a medical preparation, it is not easy to infer what the exact sense of *boot* was.

(32) ANTITODUM EMAGOGUM. þat ys to sey, **boote** or **remedye** aȝeyne euel, þat ys to sey, ledyng awey menstruel blode. (MEMT, 15th c. *AntN* (MS Fergusson 147), f. 6r)

Help and *helping*, being more frequently found than *boot* in the examined medical manuals, also seem to have had a vague medical meaning. MED suggests that both nouns expressed the sense 'medicament, medicine'. The quotations provided by the dictionary and those found in the medical material support, to some extent, this assumption, cf.:

(33) Þe second doctrine is of particuler antidoteȝ or **helpingeȝ**. (Wallner, 1425 *GCA1* (MS NY 12), 50/10)
Þu be nouȝt bolde..to vse any of **helpingez** [L auxiliorum] named euaporatyuez. (MED,?a1425 **Chauliac(1)* (MS NY 12), 165a/a)
Localez i. **helpes** [**Ch.(2)*: local medecynes] þat completeþ þe intencioun of þe augmentyng. (MED,?a1425 **Chauliac(1)* (MS NY 12), 25b/a)

Still, taking into account the fact that *help* or *helping* were mostly translations of the Latin word *auxilium* 'help, aid, assistance, support', the nouns should not be regarded as highly specialised terms for 'a medical preparation'. Rather, like perhaps in the Latin original, one can observe here a figurative use of these nouns (i.e. medical preparation seen as an aid for the ill).

3.3 Middle English adoptions of Romance terms

The most representative term in this group of nouns is *medicine* (with 1047 records), whereas the remaining five nouns (*antidote*, *confection*, *receipt*, *remedy*, *spice*) are marginally represented, at least in the sense 'a medical preparation'. What follows, is a brief discussion of the terms, with special attention to their changing senses and distribution in the analized material.

Antidote (from OF *antidote* and L *antidotum* 'a remedy against poison') was a term originally used to indicate medicines against poisonous drinks. With time, it came to mean a remedy against all kinds of poisons and later, i.e. by the time of

Galen, it became a common term to denote any medical substance counteracting various diseases (Prioreschi 2003: 592).

When the term entered English, it was used with two senses 'a medication against poisons' and 'a medication against an attack of disease'. According to MED, the earliest attestation of the term in Middle English texts dates back to the first half of the 15th century, cf.:

(34) Þe first doctrine is of vniuersale **antidotez** or helpyngez. (MED,?a1425 **Chauliac(1)* (NY 12), 6b/b)

In the analysed material, the term is found only in the translations of Guy de Chauliac's surgical texts (8 hits) and a collection of recipes known as *Antidotarium Nicholai* (5 hits). Thus, the term was not widely spread in English medical literature, and its use in the above-mentioned texts might have been the result of its transfer from the original (French and/or Latin) texts. A comparison of the two English versions of Guy de Chauliac's text on *Anatomy* (GCA1 and GCA2)[33], allows one to observe that the use of the term usually depended on the choices of a translator. Where GCA1 has the term *antidoteȝ*, the translator of GCA2 uses either *helþes* or *medicine* (cf. Table 2).

Tab. 2: General terms for 'a medical preparation' in the two English versions of Guy de Chauliac's text on Anatomy*: GCA1 and GCA2*

GCA1	GCA2
antidoteȝ or helpyngeȝ (50/9)	helþes or helpes (51/9)
antidoteȝ or helpingeȝ (50/10)	helþes (51/10)
localeȝ antidoteȝ (50/16)	helpeful medecynes (50/16)
antidoteȝ localeȝ (50/28)	stedefast helþes (51/25)
antidoteȝ localeȝ (50/32)	stedefast helþes (51/30)

In addition, in GCA1 *antidote* is accompanied (in two cases) by the Old English term *helpyngeȝ*, being some sort of explanatory term for *antidote*. This, in turn, suggests that *antidote* was not a common Middle English term, which is partly supported by the evidence found in OED. According to OED, *antidote* became a regular English term for medicaments against poisons or any diseases as late as the first half of the 16th century, cf.:

33 A comment on these two manuscripts can be found in footnote 31.

(35) Some say..that to find the **antidotum** for this disease is impossible. (OED, 1515 in Froude *Hist. Eng.* II. viii. 241)
Antidota are medicynes to be receyued within the bodye..some are gyuen agaynst poyson, some agaynst the styngyng of venemous beastes. (OED, 1543 Traheron *Vigo's Chirurg.* (1586) 431)

The noun *confection* (from OF *confeccion* and L *confectiōn-em* 'making, mixing, putting together') was first recorded in English texts in the latter half of the 14th century with the following senses: (i) 'a compound medicine or potion', (ii) 'a dish, esp. one of fruit and spices' and (iii) 'any other mixture or concoction'. The later uses of the term reveal yet another sense, i.e. (iv) 'an act of making or preparation of medicine by mixing/compounding ingredients' (MED, *confeccioun* n. and OED, *confection,* n.). In the medical material the noun is mostly found to denote sense (i) (49 records), often in fragments clarifying the type of a medical preparation, cf.:

(36) TROCISTI DIRARODON. Trocisti, þat ys to sey, a rounde **confectyoun**. (MEMT, 15th c. *AntN* (MS Ferguson 147), f. 47v)
EMPLASTRUM APOSTOLOCON. þat ys to seye, a harde **confectoun**. (MEMT, 15th c. *AntN* (MS Ferguson 147), f. 21v)

Another term, *medicine*, is an adoption of OF *medecine, medicine* 'medicine, art of healing, cure, treatment, potion' and L *medicina*. According to Charen (1951: 218), L *medicina* was used in "three substansive forms. When used with the word *ars* (art or skill) it signified the profession as we know it, medicine and sometimes surgery; with *officina* (shop) it signified the 'office' of the practitioner or the shop where his remedies were purchased; with *res* (thing, object) it signified the medicine or prescription itself".

The earliest attestations of *medicine* in Middle English texts, recorded in the 13th century, show that from the beginning the term was employed to describe any substance used in the treatment of various diseases, cf.:

(37) Þu seist þet te nis no neod **medicine**. (OED, a1225 *Ancr. R.* 178)

Also, especially in non-medical context, the term was often used figuratively and applied to mean a 'spiritual remedy; divine grace, means of grace; redemption, salvation; escape from God's wrath; a deterrent to sin, safeguard against sinning; also, mediation' (38a), or as a term relating to the solution of various social and moral problems (38b), cf.:

(38) a. Þis manere bruche mei beon ibet eft..þurh **medicine** of schrift & bireowsunge. (MED, c1230 (?a1200) *Ancr.* (Corp-C 402), 86/20)
Whe shulen into heuene blis þurh hire **medicine**; Betere is hire medycyn þen eny mede. (MED, c1325 *Nou skrynkeþ* (Hrl 2253), 30–1)

b. Was nevere such covine that couthe ordeine a **medicine** To thing which god in lawe of kind Hath set. (MED, (a1393) Gower *CA* (Frf 3), 1.30)

The noun was also used in alchemical works to denote 'a transmuting agent', i.e. "an elixir able to turn lead into gold and copper into silver." (Charen 1951: 219). Such references are found in late medieval texts on alchemy, cf.:

(39) The Elixer, a leven which is **medecyne** to all corrupe mettalls. (MED, a1500 in Singer *Cat.Alchem* 1.5 (Trin-C 1312, f.8)
Holly Alchymie..treateth of a precious **medycyne** Suche as trully maketh golde and syluer fyne. (MED, a1550 **Norton OAlch.* (BodeMus 63), 445)

In the medical texts analysed for this study, *medicine* is the noun with the highest frequency. It is recorded in compound names for medicaments e.g., *binding medicine, drying medicine, incarnative medicine, opening medicine*, etc. (178 instances; cf. chapter five, section 5.3 and Appendix B), and is used in a variety of other contexts, e.g., in the statements introducing more specific names of medical preparations (40a), in explicatory phrases to explain less familiar forms (40b), in the definitions of various specifics (40c), or in efficacy phrases that underline the effectiveness of a given medicament (40d), cf.:

(40) a. (…) and **ther be many medicynes** of that kynd as tretis emplastours oynementis pociouns that ben cleped drynkes electuaries sirupes watris oyles. (MEMT, 15th c. *ThP* (MS Sln 3489), f. 31v)
I haue putt an antidotarie of sirurgie wiþ watris, emplastris, poudris, oilis & oynementis, & **oþere dyuers medicyns in general.** (MEMT, 1475 *CHIR* (MS Wel 564), f. 10rb)
b. (…) man nor alle bodies been not like mighty to suffre and receipue þ'actions of **medicines and receiptz**. (MEMT, 15th c. *RupR* (MS Ferguson 205), 238)
Medcyn þat is called Gratia Dei. (MEMT, 1440 *LDM* (MS Thornton A.5.2), 68)
c. (…) the **medycyne callyd virtus a deo data** that knyttyth and sowdeth the tonycle ageyn yf it be brokyn. (MEMT, 1474–1499 *BG* (MS Hunter V.8.6), 98)
And þis **medycine is called Valence of scabious** for þe valow of it. (Power, 1425 *AFS* (MS Sln 6), 98/11–12)
d. [}A noþer for nassh wombe.}] Drenk tormentille ytempred wiþ hote ale made of whete. And þis is **a gode medicine** for a wounde. (MEMT, 1450–1475 *MedCh* (MS Add 34111), 139)
(…) þanne ȝe schulen haue **an heuenly medicyn** to cure perfiȝtly þis sijknesse. (MEMT, 1475 QE (MS SLN 73), 22)

Apart from sense (i) 'medical preparation' (1047 hits, 87%), the noun denoted two other senses: (ii) 'treatment/cure' (116 hits, 9%) and (iii) 'art, theory of medicine' (44 hits, 4%).

As seen in Figure 1, despite various uses and senses, the term was mostly associated with products of the pharmacist. This might be partly explained by the fact that, according to the attestations found in MED and OED, the latter senses (ii and iii) occurred in Middle English texts much later, i.e. in the first half of the 14th century (sense ii) and the end of the 14th century (sense iii). In addition, sense (ii) was more often referred to by the noun *remedy*, whereas sense (iii) was expressed by a native noun *leechcraft* (cf. the earlier discussion of *leechcraft*, section 3.1).

Fig. 1: The percentage of the occurrences of medicine *with three different senses in the analysed material*

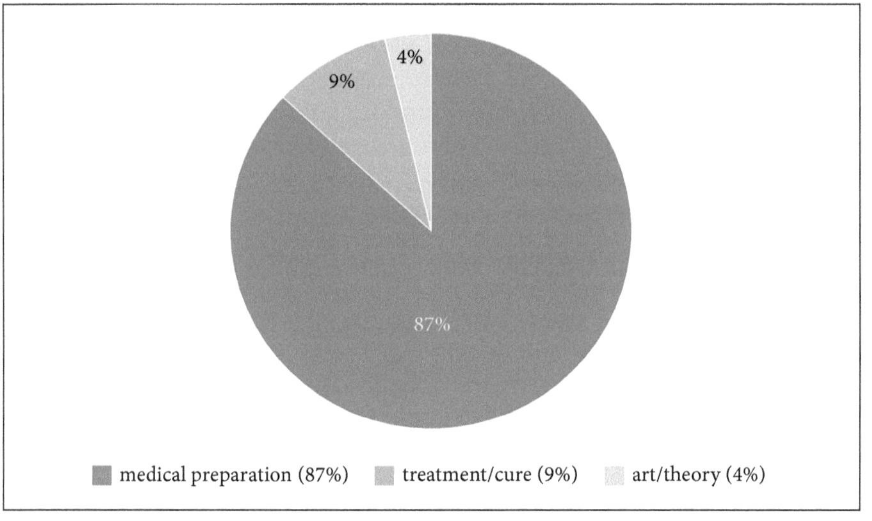

Receipt is derived from AN *recipte, receite, receyte, resceite* and from AN *receipt, recet, recept, reset, resset*. In Anglo-Norman the noun was documented with the senses (i) 'receptacle', (ii) 'receipt, receiving', (iii) 'collection (of money), money received', (iv) 'receipt (document)', (v) 'right of admission into a court; reception, act of accepting; jurisdiction', (vi) 'medical recipe' (AND, *receite* s.v., Bator — Sylwanowicz 2016: 2). The noun entered English in the 14th century and, as MED and OED reveal, was used with reference to the same ideas as in Anglo-Norman. In the medical writings analysed for the present study the noun was found only 6 times to denote 'a medical preparation', e.g.,

(41) In alle goode **resceytes** and **medicyns** amomum is ofte y-do. (MED, a1398 * Trev. *Barth.*(MS Add 27944), 214b/a)

For alle bodies been not like in taking of **receiptz**; ner þe doze nor þe porcion may not be like to euery man nor alle bodies been not like mighty to suffre and receipue þ'actions of medicines and **receiptz**. (…) And þerefore, sumtyme hit heleth men and sumtyme sleith men, þat is to seye, yeuyng of medicines and **receiptz** in thees dyuers wise wyrchen in maniere to fore seyde. (MEMT, 15th c. *RupR* (MS Ferguson 205), 238)

As seen in the examples above, the noun was often found in reduplications along with *medicine*. The use of the noun in such structures might be explained by the fact that in Middle English medical writings *receipt* was also used to denote 'a medical formula' (see 42 below). Hence, in order to avoid the confusion in identifying a particular sense ('medical preparation' or 'written formula') the compilers/translators of medical texts might have clarified the meaning of the term by using explicatory phrases such as *medicines and receiptz* (as in the examples above).

(42) Þe **receites** schal be founden in þe Antitodarye. (MED,?c1425_*Chauliac(2)*_(MS Paris angl.25), 307/9)
Þanne þou schalt do þerto turbit..in þe **resceit** tofore. (Fleischhacker, a1400 *LSC1* (MS Ashm 1396), 184/2–3)

Another term, *remedy* (OF *remedie* 'cure, remedy', L *remedium* 'antidote, cure, medicine'), is closely related to *medicine*. The noun contains the same PIE root **med*- 'to take appropriate measures, consider, advise', which later formed L *mederi* 'to heal, give medical attention to, cure'. The combination of *mederi* and a prefix *re*- 'again' formed L *remedium* 'that which heals again', the sense which was later extended to a more general sense: 'any action that corrects a wrong' (cf. Ayto 1990: 439, Haubrich 1997: 191). With this sense, i.e. 'a means of counteracting any misery or difficulty (especially evil and/or sin)', the noun entered English in the first half of the 13th century, cf.:

(43) We schulen nu speoken of þe uttre [temptation], & teachen þeo þe habbeð hire hu ha mahen wið godes grace i finde **remedie**. (MED, c1230 (?a1200) *Ancr*. (MS Corp-C 402), 94/22)
Holy bene..his **remedie** aye alle zenne. (MED, (1340) *Ayenb*. (MS Arun 57), 207/15)

The earliest attestation of the term with a medical sense is dated back to the late 14th century, when the noun was used to denote 'medical means of relief or cure' and eventually 'a medical preparation, medicament', cf.:

(44) Comyn..acordiþ to many medicynes and **remedyes** and namely of þe stomak. (MED, (a1398) **Trev. Barth*. (MS Add 27944), 220a/b)
ȝiff þes members fallen in to a peralisie, þe **remedies** owen to be leide aboute þe spondiles off þe necke. (MED,?a1425 **Chauliac(3)* (MS Htrn 95), 56b/b)

The latter sense is not frequently recorded in medical writings analysed for this study. There are only 7 hits of *remedy* denoting 'a medical preparation', cf.:

(45) Oile of roses is special **remedy** agayns brennyng and hote aposteme3, wher þat euer þai be in þe body. (Power, 1425 *AFS* (MS Sln 6), 93/34–36)
Þis oyntment wold I neuer wante for many benefete3 of it, And witte þou þat it is best **remedi** to þam þat haþe þe emoroides or þe fistule or oþer sleiyng. (Power, 1425 *AFS* (MS Sln 6), 91/10–13)

In most cases (73 hits), *remedy* has been recorded in the sense 'a method of treatment or a curative power', cf.:

(46) And þe **remedy** is þat anone þu drynke a byttir syrippe as is centory þe siruppe, and þe syruppe of wurmewode, (…). (MEMT, c1484 (1475) *DPP* (MS Takamiya 38), 150)
But þou muste contynue this **remedie** long tyme for this grete sikenes must haue long tyme of helyng yf hit haue long indurid. (MEMT, 15th c. *RupR* (MS Ferguson 205), 217)

Spice 'ingredient, sth added to the food' (from OF *espece* and L *species* 'spices, goods') is a noun whose sense varies depending on the context. It is commonly known that spices had been mostly used for culinary purposes. However, apart from food flavouring, spices were credited with marvellous healing properties and became ingredients of many medical recipes. Therefore, MED and OED suggest 'a medicine, concoction, or portion' as one of the senses of the noun *spice*, cf.:

(47) a. Somdel wiþ **spices** þat he brou3te, wiþ wicchecraft, and wiþ faire wordes, he made þe lady..mad. (MED, (a1387) Trev. *Higd.* (MS StJ-C H.1), 6/23)
b. Loue is triacle of heuene; May no synne be on him sene þat vseth þat **spise**. (MED, c1400 *PPl.B* (MS LdMisc 581), 1.147)

However, such instances of the use of the noun are mostly found in non-medical compilations and even in these samples it is not always easy to determine the exact meaning of the noun. For instance, in (47a) above *spices* could refer to various medicaments or to pepper, ginger, saffron or cinnamon, i.e. substances added to some preparations. Also, in medical compilations most records reveal that the noun denotes some condiments that, when added to a preparation, may enhance its medicinal effect. In the analysed material, there are only two records of the term as a possible referent to 'a medical preparation' in general, cf.:

(48) To make a **spyce** for þe tothewerke: Tak lij leues of sawge..and saye at þe pullynge of euer ilk a lefe a Pater noster and Aue Maria. (MED, c1440 Thrn. *Med.Bk.* (MS Thrn), 18/31)

And þerefore by þe commandement of God, ierapigra draveth corrupte humours fro þe heed, þe necke, and þe brest, and of noo membre bynethe þaym. And so I seye of other **spices** þat drauen humours fro the knees, þe legges, and þe feet (…). (MEMT, 15th c. *RupQ* (MS Ferguson 205), 115)

3.4 Distribution of the general terms denoting medical preparations in three types of texts: remedy books, surgical texts and specialised treatises[34]

The analysis of the distribution of the general terms denoting 'a medical preparation' in the three types of texts has demonstrated that not all terms were equally represented.

Medicine and *remedy* are the only nouns recorded in all types of medical texts examined for the present study. This implies that these two nouns might have been commonly recognised general terms for 'a medical preparation'. However, a closer look at the data presented in Table 3 below will reveal that this assumption holds true for *medicine*, but in case of *remedy* it proves to be incorrect. The latter term, unlike *medicine*, was not only characterised by an uneven distribution in the three types of texts but was also marginally represented (1 record, RNF: [0.3] in remedy books; 5 [1.3] in surgical texts, and 1 [0.9] in specialised treatises), at least in the sense 'a medical preparation'.

Tab. 3: The number of the occurrences of nouns denoting 'a medical preparation' in the analysed material: relative normalized frequencies (RNF per 100,000 words) are in square brackets

	Remedy books	Surgical texts	Specialised treatises
medicine	345 [96.9]	576 [150.2]	126 [112.6]
remedy	1 [0.3]	5 [1.3]	1 [0.9]
confection	31 [8.7]	18 [4.7]	0
antidote	5 [1.4]	8 [2.1]	0
receipt	5 [1.4]	0	1 [09]
help	0	6 [1.6]	0

34 There is a disproportion between the material found in the three types of medical writings. The total number of words in each collection of texts is as follows: remedy books (355 887 words), surgical texts (383 520 words), specialized treatises (111 936 words). Therefore, in the present and the following chapters, whenever the data derived from the examined collections will be compared, next to the real number of occurrences of nouns, relative normalised frequencies (RNF per 100,000 words) will also be given.

	Remedy books	Surgical texts	Specialised treatises
helping	0	3 [0.8]	0
spice	2 [0.6]	0	0
boot	1 [0.3]	0	0

Another group of nouns constitute those that were recorded in two text-types[35]. Two nouns (*antidote*, *confection*) were found in remedy books and surgical texts, whereas one, *receipt*, was recorded in remedy books and specialised treatises. All these nouns occur occasionally and are used in two or three treatises only.

The remaining four nouns (*boot*, *help*, *helping*, *spice*) are marginally represented and are peculiar to one or two treatises representing a given text type. For instance, *help*, *helping* have been found only in the translations of the surgical writings of Guy de Chauliac. Similarly, *boot* and *spice*, being recorded in remedy books, have been found in one text each.

If we consider the etymology of the nouns under discussion, their distribution in the texts also seems haphazard. However, it is possible to observe general tendencies in the selection and use of the nouns in Middle English medical writings.

Nouns of foreign origin are prevalent in all text types. Out of 7 general nouns denoting 'a medical preparation' recorded in remedy books, only 1 (*boot*) is of Germanic origin and its frequency is insignificant. A similar pattern can be observed in surgical works. Nouns of Germanic provenance (*help*, *helping*) are peripheral and, as pointed out in the previous discussion, restricted to individual texts and used as explanatory items. In specialised treatises only terms taken from foreign sources have been recorded (*medicine*, *remedy* and *receipt*). Thus, one can conclude that nouns of native origin were not widely accepted terms for 'a medical preparation'.

In the group of foreign adoptions, only *medicine* held a well-established and strong position in the field of nouns denoting 'a medical preparation'. As seen in Table 3, the noun had the highest frequency in all text-types (RNF: 96.9 in remedy books, 150.2 in surgical texts, and 112.6 in specialised treatises). Although the noun was also used to denote two other senses, i.e. 'treatment/cure' and 'art/

35 In a number of studies the term "text type" (or "text-type") is contrasted with "genre". The former is used to indicate the internal linguistic features of texts, whereas the latter is applied to classify texts according to external evidence, e.g., origin or purpose of the text (cf. Biber 1988, Taavitsainen 1997, Alonso Almeida 2008). In this work, the label "text-type" is used with reference to three groups of medical texts, i.e., remedy books, surgical texts and specialised treatises.

theory of medicine', the sense 'a medical preparation' prevailed, which can be also observed in Figure 2 below, which shows the distribution of *medicine* with its three senses in the three types of writings.

Fig. 2: The relative normalized frequencies (RNF per 100,000 words) of medicine *with three different senses in three types of medical texts*

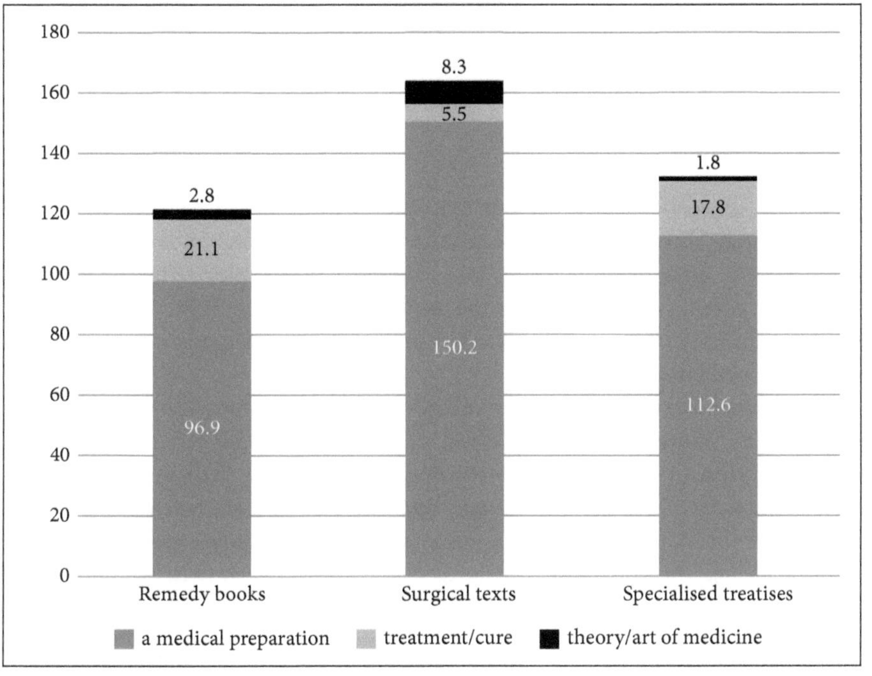

This strong position of the noun might be explained by the fact that from the moment it appeared in Middle English texts *medicine* was strongly associated with medical practice, denoting mostly preparations used in the treatment of various illnesses (cf. OED and MED n. *medicine*).

Some foreign adoptions (e.g. *remedy*, *spice*), though entered the lexicon of Middle English in approximately the same time as *medicine*, were originally used to denote more general senses, not always directly related to medical practice in its strict sense. For instance, *remedy* was first used with the sense 'counteracting any misery and difficulty' and *spice* as 'anything added to food or drink to enhance flavour'. Their use with reference to medications was recorded much later, i.e. in the second half of the 14th century. By that time, *medicine* had already been a commonly recognised medical term, which also explains why *remedy* and *spice* had a peripheral distribution, at least as nouns denoting 'a medical preparation'.

Other nouns of Romance origin (*antidote, confection, receipt*) were first documented only in the late 14th and the first decades of the 15th century. Similarly to *remedy* and *spice*, these late adoptions were originally used with a variety of senses, other than 'medicine, medicament' (cf. also the discussion in 3.3). Therefore, their use in medical compilations was scarce or even incidental, often being the choice of individual writers who either aimed to avoid repetitions or copied the forms from the original texts.

3.5 Summary

The previous sections have shown that one of the striking features of Middle English medical terminology is a number of synonymous nouns denoting the same idea(s), here general terms for 'a medical preparation'. This diversity of terms was partly a consequence of the multilingual context of the texts and their different underlying traditions of medical writing (i.e., remedy books, surgical texts and specialised treatises).

A thorough examination of the medieval medical material has revealed that at least nine nouns could have served as potential general terms for 'a medical preparation' in Middle English medical nomenclature. Within this group we have three native English items (*boot, help, helping*) and six foreign nouns, being mostly terms from Latin or French (*antidote, confection, medicine, receipt, remedy, spice*). The Germanic forms, as the analysis has shown, are marginally represented in the medical material (1/6/3 records respectively) and are used in one or two treatises only (*boot* in AntN, whereas *help* and *helping* in GCA1 and GCA2). In addition, these nouns are only found in explicatory phrases such as *boote or remedye, antidoteȝ or helpyngeȝ, localez i. helps*, which suggests that the only function of these nouns was to facilitate the understanding of probably not-yet-familiar terms. As regards the Romance examples, *medicine* is the most frequent noun (1047 records) of all general terms denoting 'a medical preparation' and is well represented in the three groups of medical writings (remedy books [RNF: 96.9], surgical texts [RNF: 150.2], and specialised treatises [RNF: 112.6]). Also, the noun is frequently used in compound forms (about 178 instances; cf. section 5.3 in chapter five and Appendix B), and in a variety of other contexts (cf. quotations under 40). Thus, it may be argued that the noun was a commonly accepted English word. The remaining nouns of Romance provenance (*antidote, confection, receipt, remedy, spice*), compared to *medicine*, seem peripheral. Their distribution in the medical texts is low (13/49/7/6/2 records respectively), and, except for *remedy*, they are restricted to one or two treatises. Their marginal position in the group of the names for 'a medical preparation' might be partly accounted for by the fact that most of them are adoptions later than *medicine*. In addition, some of them (*receipt*, *remedy*, *spice*) were also used with senses not directly related to medical practice.

Chapter four: General terms denoting dosage forms

4.1 Introduction: selection and classification

The present chapter concentrates on the names that denote the physical characteristics of medicinal preparations (e.g. *ointment*, *pill*, *syrup*). As in the previous chapter, establishing a list of nouns in question was the starting point of this chapter. The first step involved consulting earlier studies on medical terminology. Secondly, to make the list as comprehensive as possible, several dictionaries (DMVE, HTE, MED, OED) were consulted. The preliminary list of the nouns turned fairly representative and gave a general idea on what terms were commonly used in English medieval medical compilations. The final step was to read through these texts in order to (i) look for items not present in dictionaries and (ii) verify the distribution of the nouns and their frequency of use.

The above examination resulted in the body of material consisting of 40 nouns used as single terms denoting various dosage forms (cf. also tables 4, 6, 7). For practical reasons, to enhance the clarity and quality of the following discussion the nouns are grouped and dealt with according to the type of dosage forms they represent, i.e. semisolid, solid and liquid preparations[36], cf.:

(i) semisolid preparations: *anointment*, *balm*, *electuary*, *electuarium*, *emplaster*, *emplastrum*, *entrete*, *grease*, *lectuary*, *liniment*, *ointment*, *ointure*, *paste*, *plaster*, *potage*$_1$, *pultes*, *salve*, *treat*, *uncture*, *unement*, *unguent*, *unguentum*;

(ii) solid preparations: *ball*, *pellet*, *pessary*, *pill*, *pilule*, *powder*, *pulvis*, *pulver*, *suppository*, *trochisk*;

(iii) liquid preparations: *decoction*, *drink*, *liquor*, *oil*, *potion*, *potage*$_2$, *syrup*, *water*[37].

The division of pharmaceutical substances is based on modern standards (according to three types of dosage forms) in order to avoid confusion in the discussion of the terms. As the medicines have existed for ages, the pharmaceutical

---

36 In order to properly classify each noun a number of sources have been consulted, e.g., *Dorland's Medical Dictionary* (DMD), Marriott — Wilson et al. (2010), Taylor — Harding (2005), Dash — Singh — Tolman (2013), Webster (2014), Allen — Ansel (2013).

37 One of the nouns, *potage*, is recorded with reference to semisolid and liquid preparations. Hence the use of *potage*$_1$ and *potage*$_2$, respectively.

forms must have been in use ever since. And the compilers/authors of medical works were aware of different forms of preparations. While reading through the texts under study one often comes across the following statements:

(49) Here begynnyth and tellyth howe a man schal make hys **salves, playsterys, and oynementes** aftyr the forme and byddyng of mayster peers of Salarne. (MEMT, 15th c. *WBMP* (MS Med. Misc. I), 310)
In þe þridde partie I haue putt an antidotarie of sirurgie wiþ **watris, emplastris, poudris, oilis & oynementis, & oþere dyuers medicyns in general**; (MEMT, 1475 *CHIR* (MS Wel 564), 1b)

The statements as those above, usually found in the introductory parts of recipe collections, indicate that medicinal preparations were identified according to their form, i.e. salves, powders, oils. These fragments were often followed by passages concentrating on particular specifics, which were presented in the alphabetical order of their names or according to (i) ailments they were aimed to cure, and/or (ii) parts of the body they were intended for.

However, the authors and/or compilers of the texts were not always consistent in their presentations of medicinal preparations, and they frequently varied as regards the typology of medicaments. For instance, some of these writers treated plasters and ointments as related mixtures and discussed them in the same section of the text, whereas others saw them as distinct preparations. Therefore, a consistent classification of the collected names had to be invented.

Another argument for the proposed division of terms is the fact that one can easily observe the rivalry between selected terms. Within each category, we can distinguish groups of nouns related by meaning and form. For instance, the group of semisolid dosage forms contains nouns referring to 'salve-like preparations' (section 4.2.1) which only differed in their etymology (e.g. *ointment, salve, unguent, unguentum*). A thorough reading of those medical texts allows one to observe that some authors used, e.g., *ointment* or *salve*, others preferred the forms *unguent* or *unguentum*, while others mixed all the forms within the text, not always specifying that they denote the same thing. Thus, putting such nouns in groups allows a better insight into the differences of their use and distribution.

In the following sections describing particular groups of nouns, each form will be presented in terms of its etymology, the number of records in the analyzed material, as well as possible senses and uses in the examined medical material. Then, the collected data will be discussed with reference to their synonymity and possible rivalry in the three types of medical texts.

4.2 Semisolid preparations

This group includes nouns which are general terms for medicaments having "a viscosity and rigidity intermediate between that of a solid and a liquid" (CED, *semisolid* adj. and n.). Although today the term *semisolid dosage form* is usually used with reference to medicaments for treating topical ailments, i.e. those applied externally (balms, ointments, pastes), in this study the term is understood in a broader way, i.e. the focus is on the physical properties of medicaments and not on the ways of their application (externally or internally). This allows for the inclusion of, for instance, *electuary*[38] 'a medicine in which the ingredients are combined with honey or syrup to form a paste' (MED, *electuarie* n., DMD *electuary* n.), which was usually applied internally. Altogether, 22 nouns have been gathered for the category of semisolid preparations (see Table 4 below)[39].

38 Electuary is a medicament for which it is difficult to apply a clear-cut classification in terms of a pharmaceutical form. Various contexts reveal that this medicine could be grated, cut into small pieces, spread in the form of an ointment or paste, or served as a potion. Since electuary is characterised by solid and/or liquid features and both MED and OED define the noun as a preparation in a form of a paste, I have decided to include *electuary* in the discussion of semisolids.

39 Two nouns (*creme* and *smerels*) listed by the dictionaries with the sense 'salve-like preparations', i.e. semisolids, were not found in the material under study. Hence, they are not considered in this discussion. The noun *creme* has been recorded only with the sense 'the fatty part of milk, cream' (cf. MED, *creme* n.[2]) and as such was treated as an ingredient of medicinal substances. The noun *smerels* (or its clipped form *smerl*) has not been recorded at all. As OED and MED quotations show, the noun seems to have been restricted to religious practices, e.g., 'ointment used to anoint dead body or to consecrate someone'. The only medical sense of this noun, according to MED, is recorded in a non-medical text, cf.: "Þe smeryeles ne is naȝt worþ to hele þe wonde ne non oþer þing þer-huile þet þet yzen is þerinne." (MED, 1340 *Ayenb*. (MS Arun 57), 217/26).

Tab. 4: The number of the occurrences (absolute frequencies and percentage) of nouns denoting semisolid preparations in the analysed material[40]

Noun	Number of occurrences (%)	Noun	Number of occurrences (%)
anointment	8 (0.6%)	ointure	1 (0.06%)
balm	6 (0.5%)	paste	8 (0.6%)
electuarium	1 (0.06%)	plaster	555 (36.5%)
electuary	124 (8.2%)	potage$_1$	8 (0.6%)
emplaster	244 (16.2%)	pultes	9 (0.7%)
emplastrum	1 (0.06%)	salve	23 (1.5%)
entrete	27 (1.8%)	treat	16 (1.1%)
grease	2 (0.12%)	uncture	5 (0.3%)
lectuary	38 (2.5%)	unement	6 (0.5%)
liniment	3 (0.2%)	unguent	35 (2.2%)
ointment	378 (25.1%)	unguentum	8 (0.6%)

As the preparations differ in their viscosity and density, accordingly, they are discussed under the following headings: (i) ointments and salves and (ii) plasters and pastes. Due to the similarity in form and/or a relatively high degree of synonymity, some nouns will be discussed together, e.g., *ointure - uncture, plaster - emplaster - emplastrum, electuary - electuarium - letuarie, entrete - treat, unguent - unguentum.*

4.2.1 Ointments and salves

This group of nouns includes general terms denoting 'salves and/or salve-like preparations', which only differed in the bases that are used in preparing them. Thus, *anointment, grease, liniment, ointment, ointure, salve, uncture, unement, unguent, unguentum* are made using wax or greasy bases (e.g. lard, oil, wool fat, goose grease), whereas *balm* is "a salve that contains a relatively high amount of volatile oils. Upon application, it delivers a notably intense cloud of aromatic vapors." (Green 2000a: 202).

Of the 11 nouns found in the analysed material, only 1 example is of Germanic origin (*salve*), whereas the remaining 10 items are importations from

40 The number of records (in this and in the following tables in this chapter) refers to the occurrences of nouns in non-compound forms. For instance, *emplastre apostolorum, emplastre mitigatif, ointment regeneratif*, are not included in the data for *emplaster* or *ointment*. Such cases will be discussed in the section devoted to the discussion of compounds and phrases in chapter five.

Romance languages (*anointment, balm, grease, liniment, ointment, ointure, uncture, unement, unguent, unguentum*).

The noun *ointment* is the most frequently used salve-noun in medical compilations (378 occurrences), the second most frequent item is *unguent* (35 occurrences), and the third is the Old English noun *salve* with 23 occurrences. The remaining eight terms, marginally represented (altogether 39 occurrences), are shown in Figure 3 as "other", cf.:

Fig. 3: The percentage of the occurrences of nouns denoting 'salve-like preparations' in the analysed material

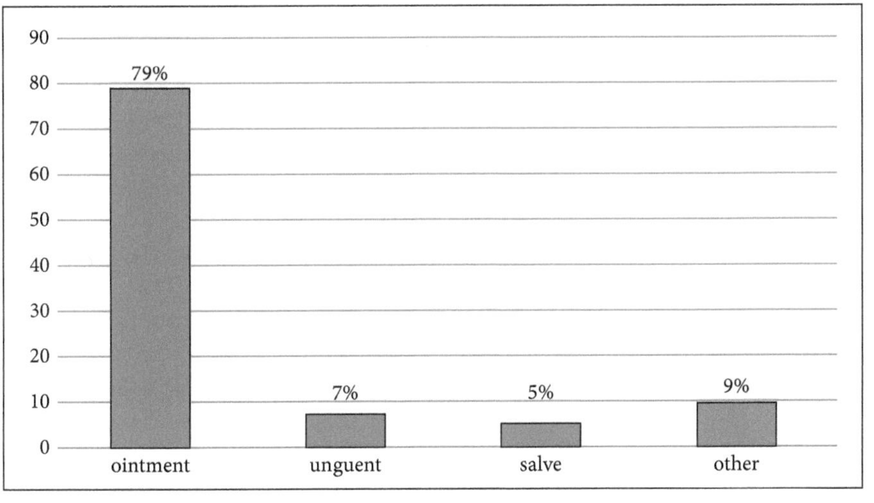

4.2.1.1 Ointment

The noun entered the lexicon of English around 1300 as a derivative of Anglo-Norman, Old French and Middle French *oinement, oignement, uniment.* Hence, the earliest texts reveal a variety of spelling forms of the noun (OED lists at least 29 variants). In later texts, that is after 1400, the noun is also recorded as a blend of *oinement* and *anointment* (cf. MED *oint(e)ment* n.), hence the forms: *oynt(e)ment, vntement* and other variant spellings, cf.:

(50) Nimeth here þis guode **oygnement**. (OED, c 1300 *St. Nicholas* (MS Laud 171), 245)
Item here is a god **oynement** for brock, (…) (MEMT, 1330 *SCC* (MS Corp-C 388), 181)
Also be þer made suche a **vntment** þat is ri3t mitigatiue. (Power, 1425 *AFS* (MS Sln 6), 12/14–15)

And thys **oyntment** is for ye scabbys good, for ye morsewe, for a felown, and for alle maner hwrtys that comyth of corrupcyon of humourys. (MEMT, 15th c. WBMP (MS Med. Misc. I), 312)
(…) and enoynt it with this **oyntement** her after ywriten (MEMT, c 1450 *LeechB1* (MS Med-L 136), 43)

From its earliest stages *ointment* was simultaneously used in two senses: (i) 'a medicinal salve prepared or used for external application' and (ii) 'a cosmetic preparation in the form of a smooth or soft paste; an ointment used to alter appearance'. In time, the noun started to denote (iii) 'sacramental or ceremonial anointing; holy oil to consecrate kings and priests' and (iv) 'an unguent used for preserving dead bodies or a grease smeared on the body or armor for protection' (cf. OED, *ointment* n. and MED, *oint(e)ment* n.). The material from MED shows that the term was also used in figurative senses such as (v) 'an act of God's grace, esp. salvation through the crucifiction of Christ' or (vi) 'a moral/spiritual virtue, the odour of sanctity'.

In the analysed material, *ointment* has been found with sense (i). The frequency of the noun is very high (approx. 378 i.e. 79% occurrences of all 'salve-like preparations'), which implies that it was a key term in the Middle English lexical field of salve-nouns[41]. This assumption is supported by the use of the noun in medical writings.

The noun is found in the discussions of types of medicaments (51a), in introductory parts to collections of recipes (*antidotaria*) (51b), or in the headings (a title and/or statement of purpose) of recipes, whose main role was to specify the ailment for which a recipe was written or indicate the type of remedy/medicament (51c), cf.:

(51) a. Compowned medicynes ben made of ij symple medicines or of more and ther be many medicynes of that kynd as tretis emplastours **oynementis** pociouns that ben cleped drynkes electuaries sirupes watris oyles. (MEMT, 15th c. *ThP* (MS Sln 3489), f. 31v)
b. (…) **oynementis**, & oþere dyuers medicyns in general; (MEMT, 1475 *CHIR* (MS Wel 564), 1b)
c. A gude **oynement for** kiles, wondes, broken bones, bolnynges, to felon & to gowte. (MEMT, 1440 *LDM* (MS Thornton A.5.2), 54)
An **oynement for** þe crampe. (MEMT, a1500 *MedW* (MSS Hrl 2378; Sln 2584; Sln 521), 82)

41 Before its introduction, that role was carried by the noun *salve* (OE *sealf*), which is also recorded in Middle English medical writings, but its frequency of use was low. For more details see the discussion on *salve* in section 4.2.1.3.

Additionally, in many recipes the noun is found as an explanatory term for salve-like specifics, mostly compound forms with L *unguentum*, cf.:

(52) And thys **oynement** ys callyd preciosum **vnguentum alabastri,** the prescyous **oynement of alabaster.** (MEMT, 1474–1499 *BG* (MS Hunter V.8.6), 63)
To make **vnguentum viridum** ffor to make **a grene oynement**. (MEMT, 15th c. *WBMP* (MS Med. Misc. I), 312)
Vnguentum fortissimum ffor to make **thys oyntment vnguentum fortissimum**. (MEMT, 15th c. *WBMP* (MS Med. Misc. I), 313)
An **oyntment** þat is called **Salus populi** is made þus: Recipe (...). (Power, 1425 *AFS* (MS Sln 6), 90//22–23)

Ointment is also found in many efficacy phrases, i.e. additional comments, usually focusing on the effectiveness of the medicament, cf.:

(53) **Þis oynement is gud for** paralisi. (MEMT, 1440 *LDM* (MS Thornton A.5.2), 66)
Þis oynement is gud for all wondis & to gedir new flesche, & fordose dede flesche. (MEMT, 1440 *LDM* (MS Thornton A.5.2), 73)
Ffor thys maner of pannycle ys curyd wyth **thys precious oynement.** (MEMT, 1474–1499 *BG* (MS Hunter V.8.6), 63)

In many passages of the analysed material we find instances where the noun *ointment* is used to specify precisely the dosage form a medicament should have. Such instances have been recorded in the recipes for preparations other than salves, e.g., pastes. Thus, as the examples below show, a mixture has to be first prepared in the form of an ointment before other ingredients are added in order to make a thicker preparation:

(54) And stampe them wele togeddyr wyth womans mylke, mollifi yt **tyl yt be as an oynement**, wherof make a plaster and lay it to the sore. (MEMT, 1474–1499 *BG* (MS Hunter V.8.6), 77)
For to defend þat no wykkyd mater draw to no wound. Tak a vnce off bool armoniak and (...) stere it to-geder, and so do lytyl and lytyl **tyl it be standyng þykke as an oynement;** and sprede it on a cloþe and ley it on, an handbrede a-boue þe wound, ouere þe sore, tyl it be hoole. (MEMT, a1500 *MedW* (MSS Hrl 2378; Sln 2584; Sln 521), 138)

4.2.1.2 Unguent, unguentum

Unguent is a derivative of L *unguentum* 'ointment', which according to OED and MED, entered English in the 15th century, both in medical and non-medical contexts, cf.:

(55) **Vnguent** is a þing vnctuous, not fluide, i. rynnyng, bot abiding, And þai be made after common doctrine. (MED, a1425 *Chauliac (1)* (NY 12), 167a/a]

Or madifie hit so in oil lauryne, Let drie hem, sowe hem, vp by oon assent They wol, and haue odour like her **vnguent**. (OED, c1440 *Pallad. On Husb.* IV. 147)

In the analysed material *unguent*, as a simple lexical unit, is rare and seemingly restricted to particular texts, mostly surgical writings. Of the 35 records found in the material under study, 21 instances of the noun are present in the translations of Guy de Chauliac's surgical treatises. The use of *unguent* in these texts, instead of a more common noun *ointment*, might be the choice of the translator(s) who wanted to be closer to the original version of the text. For instance, two 15th century translations of Guy de Chauliac's *Anatomy* (GCA1 and GCA2) reveal how translators often varied in their choice(s) of terms[42]. In GCA1 we will find *unguent*, whereas the author of GCA2 uses *ointment*, cf. also Table 5 below.

Tab. 5: The use of references to salve-*nouns in the two English versions of Guy de Chauliac's text on* Anatomy*: GCA1 and GCA2*

	GCA1	GCA2
1.	10/10–12 to bere with hym .5. **vnguents** .s. basilicon for to maturatiue, vnguentum *Apostolorum* to Mundificatiue. vnguentum aureum to incarnatyue, vnguentum album to consolidatiue, Dialteam to dulcoratiue.	11/9–12 bere wiþ hym fyue **oynementes**, þat is to wite, basilicon to maturynge, vnguentum *apostolorum* to clensynge and mundefieng, vnguentum aureum for to make flesche / vnguentum album to knyttynge / & dialteam to make swete
2.	20/19–20 with **vnguents** & with swete emplasteres	21/25 wiþ swete **oynementis** and emplastres
3.	50/24 How **vnguentes** bene made.	51/23 how **oynementis** beþ made

Interestingly, example 1 in GCA2 confirms the assumption proposed in section 4.2.1.1 that the noun *ointment* might have been treated as a Middle English key term denoting salve-like preparations.

As regards L *unguentum*, it is not as common as its derivative *unguent* and all its records (8 hits) used as a simple term for 'ointment' have been documented only in surgical and specialised works (cf. examples under 56 below), which suggests that it might have been regarded as a highly technical term. *Unguentum* is much more frequent (69 records, cf. Appendix B) in compound forms such as *unguentum apostolorum*, *unguentum aureum*, *unguentum album*, i.e. names for more specific ointments[43].

42 For more details see Sylwanowicz (2009).

43 See also the discussion on compounds and phrases in chapter five.

(56) At laste be þer putte storax, And be þer made **vnguentum**, Of þe which þe ceruix.i. paxwax, þe necke [&] þe chyne and al þe body be anoynted atuix .2. fireȝ. (Wallner, 1425 *GCW* (MS NY 12), 44/1–4)
And to þe same entensioun *Auicen* enditeþ þis medicyne expert, & *Brune* graunteþ it[:] Recipe draganti rubei (…), be þer made **vnguentum**. (Wallner, 1425 *GCU* (MS NY 12), 26/17–20)
Vnguentum is maad of .. oile..wex & .. of þingis þat þin oynement schal serue þerfore. (Fleischhacker, a1400 *LSC1* (MS Ashm 1396), 330/22–24)
The next day folowyng all [{h{]is soris was anoynted with this **unguentum**. Re oleti ross butter ana. oz. j. jous of femiterre planten (…). (MEMT, 15th/16th c. *TTP* (MS Sln 389), 464)

4.2.1.3 Salve[44]

Salve is the only Germanic item (derived from West Germanic **salƀo-* 'oily substance', cf. Old Saxon *salba*, Middle Dutch *salve*, Dutch *zalf*, Old High German *salba*, and German *Salbe* 'ointment') in the group of Middle English nouns denoting 'salve-like preparations'. According to OED and MED, this item was originally used as a term denoting solely a medicinal mixture that was applied to wounds or sores. This sense was found in both, medical and non-medical context, cf.:

(57) *Malagma*, **salb**. (OED, a700 *Epinal Gloss*, 635)
Genim þas yclan wyrte, wyrc to **salfe**. (OED, c1000 *Sax. Leechd*. I. 110)
Wiþ innoþes stirunga, nim þeos wyrt, wyrc to **sealue**, le3e to þan innoþes sare. (MED, c1150 *Hrl.HApul*.(MS Hrl 6258B), 106.76/3)
Ure lauerdes sonde, þe bochte **salue**..to healen hire tittes. (OED, c1225 *Ancrene Riwle* (MS Cleo. C.vi),272)

A thorough reading of Old English collections of medical texts confirms that originally *salve* was the commonest Anglo-Saxon noun used for 'salve-like preparations'. *Leechbook* (Cockayne 1864–1866) and the Old English versions of *Herbarium* and *Medicina de Quadripedibus* (de Vriend 1984) contain 175 records of the term, including 63 records in compound forms with *salve* (OE *sealf*) as a head noun, e.g., *bæþsealf, blacansealfe, dolgsealf, driȝesealf, eaȝsealf, earsealf, ȝodsealf, heafod sealf, muþsealf, onlecȝende sealf, smeresealf, toþsealf, weaxsealf*. Other Old English terms, according to TOE and HTE, used with the same reference included: *sape, sealfcynn, smerenes, smirenes, smirung, teafor, smerles* (<*smirels*). Many of these terms are not found in Old English medical texts or,

44 This section is partly based on Sylwanowicz 2014b; the material has been revised and extended.

compared with *salve*, their frequency is underrepresented (e.g. only 5 records of *smirung*, and 2 records of *smerenes*).

Although in Middle English writings *salve* was mainly employed with reference to bodily ailments, with time, i.e. in the 13th century, the noun developed a figurative meaning: 'a spiritual or religious remedy', cf.:

(58) Iesumm, Mann kinne **sawle sallfe**…Him hafe we nun fundenn. (OED, c1200 *Ormulum* (Burchfield transcript), I. 13489)
Prude Salue is ed modnesse. (OED, c1225 (1200) *Ancrene Riwle* (MS Cleo. C.vi), 202)

Later, i.e. 14th–15th century, works show that the noun was more commonly used with the second sense, also as an epithet of the Virgin Mary, e.g., "Haile, swete **salue** for al maner sare." (OED, a 1500 *Heil be þou marie þe* (Dub 516)). This implies that at some point the noun might have been confused with or treated as a form derived from the 14th century verb *salue* (from L *salutare* 'to greet' and *salus* 'greeting, good health'), cf. *Salue Regina.* Both terms are recorded with the same spelling and, as the MED reveals, the Latin term is also found as a noun, e.g., "Alle þat wylle.. þis **salue** singe ore say Wit deuocyon..þaire aduokete I þe make." (MED, a1400 *Monk Sees Virg.* MS Eg 2810). Thus, *salve* 'ointment' might not have been treated as a scholarly term by Middle English medical compilers who, as the texts reveal, more often turned to foreign terms, i.e. *ointment* or *unguent* (cf. also Tables 8 and 9 that list the number of the occurrences of nouns in the three types of medical texts, section 4.5). This assumption can be supported by the fact that of the documented 23 records of the noun *salve* 21 instances are found only in texts that are classified as remedy books, i.e. texts representing longer tradition of medical writing, dating back to Old English, but characterised as less scholarly, often incorporating non-learned medicine.

In the analysed corpus, apart from a general sense 'salve' (59a), the noun seems to have been restricted to denote a medicinal application for wounds (59b) or sores (59c).

(59) a. Here begynnes makyng of **salues**, tretys, oynementys good and trewe, without fayle; or to make **salue**. (Henslow, a1500 *HMW* (MSS Hrl 2378; Sln 2584; Sln 521), 117/17–18)
Here bygynnes þe maner to mak **salues** & entretis & drynkes & cyroyns to wondis (MEMT, 1440 *LDM* (MS Thornton A.5.2), 69)
b. An oþer **salue** to wonde on þe body. (MEMT, 1440 *LDM* (MS Thornton A.5.2), 70)
A gud **salue** for wondis. (MEMT, 1440 *LDM* (MS Thornton A.5.2), 73)
(…) close þe wound with **selue**. (Henslow, a1500 *HMW* (MSS Hrl 2378; Sln 2584; Sln 521) 59/10–11)

c. A **Salve** for all soorys. Also for to make a **connyng salve for all sorys**. (MEMT, 15th c. *WBMP* (MS Med. Misc. I), 317)

4.2.1.4 Peripheral nouns: anointment, balm, grease, liniment, ointure, uncture, unement

This section presents salve-nouns whose frequency in the analysed material is relatively low (cf. Table 4)[45], and consequently these nouns are not discussed in separate sections. Some of them (*grease, liniment, ointure, uncture, unement*, cf. also Table 10 in section 4.5) are found in only one of the texts under study, which suggests their peripheral character in medical lexis. In addition, three nouns (*balm, grease, liniment*) were originally associated with senses other than 'medicinal salve, ointment'.

Anointment

The noun is derived from OF *enointen* (v.) which appeared in English in the first half of the 14th century and, according to OED, partially replaced OE *smerian* 'smear', "as a more refined and specialised synonym" (OED, *anoint* v.). The verb developed various senses relating to an 'act of applying oil or ointment'. Although the verb is recorded in a medical context with the sense 'to apply medicine or a healing unguent', most quotations provided by MED reveal that the verb was frequently used in a religious context with the senses: (i) 'to anoint/consecrate (a king, priest, etc.)', (ii) 'to bless or sanctify (someone) as with a sacrament', (iii) 'to embalm a dead body'. This partly explains the low frequency of its derivative noun *anointment* in the medical writings studied for the present work (8 records, cf. Table 4). In addition, it is possible that the noun might have been confused with a more common noun *ointment*, cf.:

(60) Also for to make a **noyntement** for brenyg [\f. 13v\] of ye fyre. Take rode and brene yt all to poudyr aschys. (…) For in trwthe thys **oynement** hath be prevyd. (MEMT, 15th c. *WBMP* (MS Med. Misc. I), 314)
Also for to make **an oynement** for to put a weye ye saws flewme in the vyssage. (MEMT, 15th c. *WBMP* (MS Med. Misc. I), 314)
Here is makyng of **anoynement** sanatif. Tak þe same herbes þat goþ to saue & worche hem (…) do saue to þis **oynement**. (Alonso, a1400 *Recipes* (MS Hunter 185), 97/23–26)

45 The form *unguentum*, whose frequency in the examined material is also low, is discussed together with *unguent* due to the similarity in form and their high degree of synonimity.

Taking into account the examples above it is difficult to state, without doubt, whether their users had in mind *anoyntment*, *nointment* or *an oyntment* (this last example is the most common variant in the examined medical writings). Thus, was the use of different forms in the same recipe an intended choice or was it a scribal error? Following OED, a similar confusion occurred in the case of the verb *anoint* which was analysed phonetically as *a* + *noint*, yielding the aphetized form *noint,* hence *nointment.* In the medical material, such examples are rare and have little influence on the overall data collected for the present study.

Balm

The noun developed from OF *baume, basme* (from L *balsamum* 'aromatic oleoresin from a balsam tree'). The earliest records reveal that originally the form of the noun followed a French pattern, hence ME *baum(e), bawm(e), basme, bame.* In later texts, we can observe a gradual alteration of the form to *balsme, bawlsme, bawlme* and eventually *balm.* According to OED (*balm* n.), this change was influenced by L *bal-*.

The earliest attestations of the noun in the written sources date back to the first half of the 13th century. At that time, the noun was used with the following senses: (i) 'the aromatic oleoresin of the balm of Gilead and other shrubs of the genus Commiphora; the shrub or tree yielding balsam' and (ii) 'an embalming ointment or fluid' (MED, *baume* n.). Later texts, from the end of the 14th century, reveal a sense reflecting the curative properties of the substance: (iii) 'aromatic ointment used for soothing pain or healing wounds' (cf. MED and OED). According to OED, the noun was also used to denote (iv) 'some fragrant herbs'.

The analysed corpus contains only 6 records of the noun with reference to sense (iii), either as an external (61a) or internal (61b) preparation, cf.:

(61) a. For to maken **baume.** Take herbe Ion to-forn the fest of seynt Iohn Baptist, and grynd it in a morter (…). For to receyvett the **baume**, and do so with alle thy balles and thanne put it in a clene glas vessell; and wete wel that it hath the same vertu that the other **baume** hath, but it ne dureth in þe vertu but iii ȝeer. (MEMT, a1500 *MedW* (MSS Hrl 2378), 78)
Stronge dissolutiues ben (…) **bawme** þat is an onyment (…). (Getz, a1475 *GA* (MS Wel 537), 37/20–21)
(…) for hit ys worþe **baume** for any maner of malady of þe sore yen. (Heinrich, c1450 *HRec* (MS Add 33996), 102/21)
b. Oþer medicynes þer be weche if a woman drinke þer of þei wyll make þem to hafe purgacioun or delyuer hyre of a ded childe if þer is ony with yn hyre. As **bawme** y dronke (…). (Hallaert, a1500 *SW1* (MS Yale-M 47), 37/190–192)

Other instances (33 occurrences), where *balm* is listed as an ingredient for some medicinal preparation, reflect senses (i) and (iv). This suggests that *balm* as 'salve' had a marginal position in the group of Middle English salve-like preparations.

Grease

Grease, from OF *gre(i)sse* 'grease, fat' and L **crassia* '(melted) animal fat', appeared in English in the late 13th century (OED, *grease* n.). In the medical material, the noun is mostly recorded as an ingredient of various preparations (usually salves or pastes) and is often accompanied by a name of the animal whose fat is used in preparing the substances, e.g., *swynes grece*, *hors grece*, *bores grece*, *fox grece*, *hennes grece*, etc. According to MED, the noun denoted also 'unguent, ointment' and this use of the noun is recorded only 2 times in the analysed material. These instances have been found in one text, cf.:

(62) Stampe hyt..wel as hyt ys seyde byfore in þe **greces** of woundes. (Heinrich, c1450 *HRec* (MS Add 33996), 227/20)
(…) wel stampe hyt wyþ þe forseyd **greces**. (Heinrich, c1450 *HRec* (MS Add 33996), 227/33)

Liniment

The earliest records of the noun, derived from L *linimentum* 'a soft ointment', date back to the first half of the 15th century and, according to OED and MED, denoted (i) 'ointment, salve' or in general (ii) 'something used for smearing or anointing'. *Liniment* was not a very common noun at that time, which is confirmed by a handful of quotations provided by OED and MED. In the medical corpus studied for the present work the noun has been found only in the writings of Guy de Chauliac (3 occurrences), cf.:

(63) And be made of hem a **liniment**. (Wallner, 1425 *GCU* (MS NY 12), 26/22)
(…) & be þer made a **linyment** or vngtment (…). (Wallner, 1425 *GCU* (MS NY 12), 61/10)
I vsed a **liniment** or vnguent praised of Heben Mesue in passionȝ of þe hert, with which is anoynted þe necke, þe backe & þe membreȝ yhurt. (Wallner, 1425 *GCW* (MS NY 12), 48/7–9)

In the MED are found 3 more instances of the term in the work by the same author, cf.:

(64) Bete þam al smal..& distempre þam with þe succo of semperviue..and be þer made a **liniment** [**Ch.(2)*: emplastrynge; L linimentum]. (MED,?a1425 **Chauliac(1)* (NY 12), 25b/a)

Be þer made a **liniment**, i. oyntment, of which be he epithimated in þe baþ & abide stille. (MED,?a1425 *Chauliac(1)* (NY 12), 115a/b)
Also þer bene many oþer manerez of componyng helpes as..**linimentes**, i. anoyntyngez. (MED,?a1425 *Chauliac(1)* (NY 12), 167b/a)

Thus, as the examples reveal, *liniment* seems peripheral and probably not well known as in most cases (cf. examples above) the noun is explained by other, more common salve-nouns, e.g., *unguent*, *ointment*. It is highly possible that translator(s) merely copied the term from the original text and, to make sure it would be well understood, provided some explanation, which was a common practice in Middle English medical writings.

Ointure and *uncture*

Both nouns, derived from the same Latin source, entered English around 1400, hence they are discussed together. *Ointure* was derived from AN *oynture* and MF *ointure* (both from L *unctura* 'ointure'), whereas *uncture* was directly taken from a Latin form. In the analysed material, both forms are recorded only in two translations of Lanfranc's *Science of Surgery* (1 record of *ointure* in LSC1 and 5 of *uncture* in LSC2), cf.:

(65) a. I dide ofte tymes þe same medicyn & þe same **oynture**. (Fleischhacker, a1400 *LSC1* (MS Ashm 1396), 103/6–7)
b. (…) y dede efte sonys þe same medycine & þe same **vncture**. (Fleischhacker, a1450 *LSC2* (MS Add 12056), 103/25–26)
c. ȝif a posteme were for þe prikynge of a synwe, ne leye noȝt þereto þis potage maturatyff, but wyt þe **vncture** of oyle of roses (…). (Fleischhacker, a1450 *LSC2* (MS Add 12056), 56/38–39)

The single occurrence of *ointure,* which in a later translation (LSC2) is rendered as *uncture* (65b), supports one of the assumptions provided by the editors of OED, which considers also possible that *ointure* is an alteration of *uncture* after *oint* (OED, *ointure* n.). The examples above reveal that the noun *uncture* was not only used to denote 'ointment, salve' but also 'the act of the application of a healing oil' (MED, *enointure* n., cf. example 65c). This and the fact that the noun seems restricted to one text only implies that it was a marginal noun in the lexical field of medical salve-nouns.

Unement

Although in MED and OED the noun is treated as an alternative form of *ointment* (cf. MED *oinement* n. and OED *ointment* n.), in DMVE the noun has its own entry. Derived from OF *unnement* and AN *u(y)nemet*, *uniment* it entered English with the sense 'ointment, greasy preparation mixed with some medicament' (DMVE, *unement* n.). In the examined material, it was recorded in the 14th century collection of medical recipes written in English, French or Latin. The noun is probably a direct adoption of a Romance form, as it has been found 7 times in the recipes written in French (as *unement*, cf. examples under 66a), and 6 times in the recipes documented in English (as *vnement*, examples under 66b)[46], cf.:

(66) a. Item le sindre de vine pernez e os de beste e veut oynt de porck, si fettes **unement** e oynez le chef.viii. joures ou.ix. (MEMT, 1330 *FCC* (MS Corp-C 388), 100)
Item **unement** prove pur macle e teye: Mettez eycile mut (…). (MEMT, 1330 *FCC* (MS Corp-C 388), 103)
b. Item a god **vnement** for alle gutes: Tack an owele and do of þe (…). (MEMT, 1330 *SCC* (MS Corp-C 388), 175)
For sausefleme visage: Tack þe rote of horshelin and (…) mack **vnement** and gres þe visage. (MEMT, 1330 *FCC* (MS Corp-C 388), 108)

4.2.2 Plasters and pastes

This group of semisolid preparations also comprises 11 forms: *emplaster*, *emplastrum*, *electuary*, *electuarium*, *entrete*, *lectuary*, *paste*, *plaster*, *potage*$_1$, *pultes*, *treat*, all of which denote 'paste-like mixtures for healing and/or cosmetic purposes'. These mixtures, compared with salves, are characterised by much higher viscosity and often require heating before their application. Usually these preparations were applied only topically (*emplaster*, *emplastrum*, *entrete*, *plaster*, *treat*) but some of them could be taken internally (*paste*, *electuary*, *electuarium*, *lectuary*, *potage*$_1$, *pultis*).

Plaster (555 occurrences), *emplaster* (244 occurrences) and *electuary* (124 occurrences) are the commonest items in this group of nouns, and these three together represent 90% of all instances of 'paste-like mixtures'. The next group of nouns (*entrete*, *lectuary*, *treat*) constitutes only 8% of all terms, and thus their influence on the lexical field seems insignificant. Likewise, the remaining three nouns (*paste*, *potage*$_1$, *pultes*) are marginally represented (about 2%), and these three nouns are shown in Figure 4 as "other".

46 In the present study only the records of *unement* documented in Middle English recipes are taken into account. The English fragments with 6 records of *vnement* are not translations of the French recipes with the 7 records of *unement*. These are different recipes, some in French and some in English, that are gathered in one collection.

Fig. 4: The percentage of the occurrences of nouns denoting 'paste-like preparations' in the analysed material

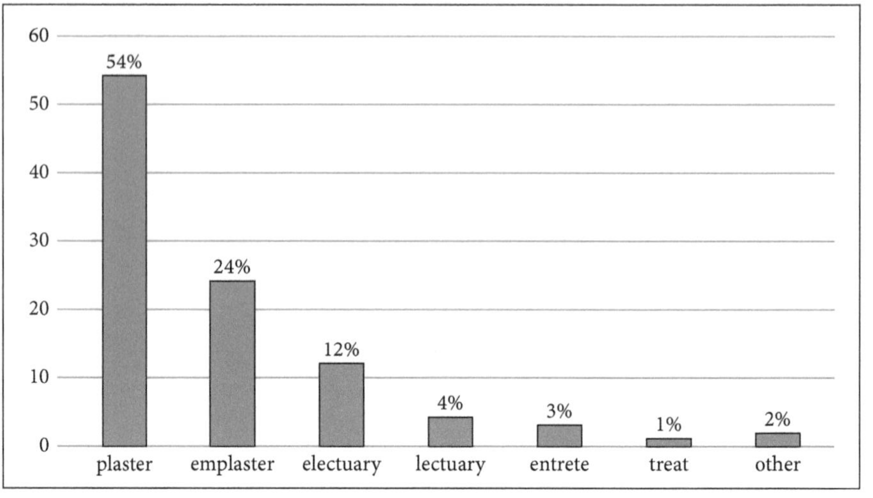

4.2.2.1 Plaster, emplaster, emplastrum

Plaster is the only noun within this category which was used as early as Old English[47]. The noun developed from L *plastrum*, a shortened form of L *emplastrum* 'plaster' (OED, *plaster* n.). In Old English medical texts the term is used only 4 times, which makes it a marginal term in a group of Old English semisolid preparations[48].

The examples in MED and OED demonstrate that the noun gained on importance, at least in the medical sense, at the beginning of the 14th century. This is also evidenced by the text corpus analysed for this study. In the earliest medical writings (FCC and SCC)[49], dated back to 1330, the noun has 30 records (about 5% of all *plaster* records in the examined Middle English medical texts).

47 According to TOE, *plaster* was not the only Old English term denoting 'some medicinal paste-like substance applied on the skin'. TOE lists the following Old English nouns denoting 'plaster, poultice': *clām, cliþa, flacg, flyne, lǣcedōmes, onlegen, plaster, sweþung* (TOE, 02.08.12.02.05.03).

48 Other terms found in Old English medical texts include *clām* (5 occurrences), *cliþa* (17 occurrences) and *onlegen* (16 occurrences).

49 These texts are included in the Appendix to MEMT.

In the analysed material, the noun is found in the headings of recipes (67a), in fragments specifying a dosage form of a given preparation (67b) or as an explanatory term for L *emplastrum* (67c), cf.:

(67) a. (…) it is conteynyd in þe boke þat I made þe of medycynys compounyd and of crafty watrys and drynkys, in confecte vnguentys and **plastrys** (…). (MEMT, c1484 (1475) *DPP* (MS Takamiya 38), 167)
A plaster for wondis. (MEMT, 1440 *LDM* (MS Thornton A.5.2), 74)
A plastyr for a sor hede. (MEMT, a1500 *MedW* (MSS Hrl 2378), 82)

b. (…) and ley hit above **in manere of a plaster**, and thys ys the most perfygthe mater that we prove. (MEMT, 15th c. *AW* (MS Hrl 2381), 37)
and also ȝef yt be put **on þe maner of a plastere** on þe temples (…). (MEMT, 15th c. *AntN* (MS Ferguson 147), f. 29r)

c. **Emplastrum Oxiorociu.** Also here be the makyng of playstrys, and fyrste to make yis **plastyr Oxiorocin**. (MEMT, 15th c. *WBMP* (MS Med. Misc. I), 314)
Emplastyr Turbentyne. Also for to make **thys playstyr Turbentyn**. (MEMT, 15th c. *WBMP* (MS Med. Misc. I), 314)

Additionally, there are a few examples of a specific use of the noun (cf. 68). Two interpretations are possible: (i) a number of plasters that should be used (68a), or (ii) a given plaster should be applied a number of times in order to heal the patient (68b), cf.:

(68) a. (…) he schal be hole within iij **plastres**. (MEMT, c1450 *JBurg* (MS Sln 2320), 216)

b. (…) and wyt-yn IX **plastyris** he schall be hole. (MEMT, c1450 *JBurg* (MS Sln 2320), 218)

The noun *plaster* often co-occurs with its synonym, *emplaster* (from OF *emplastre* and its etymon L *emplastrum*). The earliest records of *emplaster* are attested in the written sources dated back to the end of the 14th century and since then the noun had been in common use for 'a medicinal preparation in the form of a sticky paste; usually applied to the skin on piece of linen or leather'. Unlike *plaster*, which was also used in a building context 'a composition of lime, sand, etc., for plastering walls or other surfaces' (MED, *plastre* n.), *emplaster* entered English with medical sense only.

In the analysed material *emplaster* is fairly well represented (244 occurrences, 24% of all plaster-like terms), especially in surgical texts (cf. section 4.5). In the medical writings the noun is often used interchangeably with *plaster*, an alternative form when referring to this medical preparation, cf.:

(69) A noþer. Tak þe iuse of ribwort, and þe white of a neye, et ryemele, and mak a past and þer of a **plastre**, (…) and afterwardes lege to a noþer **emplastre** til þat it be hole, et þis is yprouid. (MEMT, 1450–1475 *MedCh* (MS Add 34111), 132)

As regards *emplastrum*, it is documented as a single term only once, in the surgical writing (LSC1), where the author provides an explanation of the term (cf. 70 below). The form is much more common in compound forms, being names of specific preparations, e.g., *emplastrum apostolicon, emplastrum attractivum, emplastrum nerval, emplastrum rubeum*, etc. (30 records, cf. Appendix B).

(70) **Emplastrum** is seide, whanne manie diuers þingis, as poudris and gummis & fatnessis, wex, talow, & oile ben soden togidere til þei bicome hard, & maad in gobetis & kept. & þan it schal be maad abrood vpon leþir, & leid vpon þe place (…). (Fleischhacker, a1400 LSC1 (MS Add 12056) 331/1–5)

4.2.2.2 Electuary, electuarium, lectuary

Electuary comes from L *electuarium*, which, according to OED (*electuary* n.), was probably a corrupt derivative of Gk. ἐκλεἰκτον (*ekleikton*, 'a medicine which is licked away'). This way of application (i.e. licking) of *electuary*, is prescribed in the Hippocratic Corpus[50] which says that "[t]he patient should lick the remedy along with honey" (after Pocuca — Stupar 2006: 50). In later medical documents licking is no longer advised as an application form.

In Middle English medical writings *electuary* appeared in the late 14th century and soon became a very common term (124 records)[51] used with the sense 'a medicinal preparation in which the ingredients are combined with honey or syrup to form a paste', which was taken orally and in small quantities, cf.:

(71) Bete all thyes to powder and sars þem and confete hem togedder wyth claryfyed hony, and make **electuarye**. And of thys lete the pacyent resceyue yn the mornyng fastyng <u>the quantite of a good chasteyn or of a walnot,</u> and at eue to bed-ward as much. (MEMT, 1474–1499 *BG* (MS Hunter V.8.6), 57)

Lectuary 'a medicine in a form of a paste', from OF *letuaire* (an aphetic form of L *electuarium*), appeared in English texts much earlier (the first half of the 13th century) than *electuary*. And this form has been found (5 records) in the earliest medical texts (FCC and SCC) of the analysed material, cf.:

(72) þerto is þis **letuarie** god and is cald laxatiue for þe stomack confortatiue for þe heued: Tac ceve a god partie (…) and do it in newe scured panne and dittet os it were a **letuarie**. (MEMT, 1330 *FCC* (MS Corp-C 388), 121)

50 The oldest Ancient Greek collection of medical works (Porter 2001: 56).

51 According to Pocuca — Stupar (2006: 50) in one text, i.e. *Antidotarium Nicholai* there are described at least 75 different *electuaria* out of 142 remedies (though only five are listed by their name). See also the discussion of specifics in chapter five.

Letuarie for þat nowit may wel eten: Tack þe ious of þe fenyl (…). (MEMT, 1330 *SCC* (MS Corp-C 388), 167)
Letuarie. God **letuarie** agayn al manere eueles for hoes, for þe brest, (…). (MEMT, 1330 *SCC* (MS Corp-C 388), 167)

As the examples above show, from the beginning the noun denoted a universal medical preparation used to heal various ailments and parts of the body. In later texts, the noun is recorded 33 times, usually as an explanatory term for the names of specifics (73a) or as a term indicating a pharmaceutical form of a preparation (73b), cf.:

(73) a. ELECTUARIUM AD RESTURACIONEM HUMIDITATES. þat ys to seye a **lectuarye** to restorynge of humydite. (MEMT, 15th c. *AntN* (MS Ferguson 147), f. 25r)
b. (…) distemprie the cassia fustula and þe tamaryndes, and so confecte yt on þe maner of a **lectuarye**. (MEMT, 15th c. *AntN* (MS Ferguson 147), f. 25v)

As regards L *electuarium*, it is documented as a single term only once in an English translation of the treatise on syphilis (TTP)[52]. As it can be seen in the quotation below, the Latin form is used in the heading (title/statement of purpose) of the recipe, whereas in the main body of the text a more familiar form (*electuary*) is used, cf.:

(74) **Electuarium** comforting the hert & the brayn & the liver in this cause. Re specierum diarodon abbtis dr. j +s zuccar (…). And of **this electuary** the patient shall use it in morsells viij in noumbre and by godds grace this shall suffice. (MEMT, 15th/16th c. *TTP* (MS Sln 389), 173)

Electuarium is more common (17 records, cf. Appendix B) in the names of specifics, e.g., *electuarium de succo rosarum, electuarium ducis, electuarium dulce, electuarium patris, electuarium pluris*, etc.

4.2.2.3 Entrete, treat

Entrete and its aphetic form *treat*, from OF *entrait* and *trait*, appeared in English writings simultaneously (around 1400) with the sense 'a medicinal plaster'. The preparations named by these two nouns, unlike other paste-like medicaments, often had wax or oil of roses as the main ingredients, cf.:

52 *The tretece of the pokkis* is a fragmentary translation of Latin original by Gaspar Torrella (*Tractatus cum consillis contra pudendrugram seu morbum gallicum*) dated back to the end of the 15th century. According to the editors of MEMT, it is the earliest English treatise on syphilis. For more see, e.g., Zimmerman (1937).

(75) (…) an **entreet** maad of ij parties of whiȝt rosyn, & oon partie of wex moltun togidere. (Fleischhacker, a1400 *LSC1* (MS Ashm 1396), 132/3–5)
(…) & aboue al þis I leie on a **treet** of whiȝt rosyn. (Fleischhacker, a1400 *LSC1* (MS Ashm 1396), 135/18)

In the analysed material, the two terms do not differ much in their frequency of use (*entrete* 27 records, *treat* 16 records) and are often used interchangeably in the same text or passage, cf.:

(76) þanne take out þe **trete**, &~ kerue hit, 3ef þou wolt; for þis ys good **entret** &~ kyndely made on warantyse. (Heinrich, c1450 *HRec* (MS Add 33996), 83/10–11)
For to make **a good entret**. Tak iij quartrons of spaynyssch code (…). (Alonso, a1400 *Recipes* (MS Hunter 185), 96/23)
Also for **tret** j made with herbes. Tak beteyne, verueyne, (…). (Alonso, a1400 *Recipes* (MS Hunter 185), 96/31)

4.2.2.4 Peripheral nouns: potage$_1$, pultes, paste

The nouns discussed in this section are categorised as peripheral due to a very small number of occurrences (altogether 2% of all paste-like nouns). In addition, two of these nouns (*potage*$_1$ and *pultes*) have been found in only one text.

Potage$_1$

Potage, from OF *potage, pottage*, entered English in the 13th century with the sense (i) 'a thick soup or stew, variously with or without meat; a soup containing leguminous vegetables: beans, peas, lentils, etc.;' (MED, *potage* n.). In the 15th century, according to MED and OED, the noun was also recorded with the sense (ii) 'poultice', i.e. a paste-like preparation applied to the skin'. As the noun has been identified in the medical material with both senses it has been categorised in two separate groups: sense (i) in liquids (*potage*$_2$) and sense (ii) in semisolids (*potage*$_1$). This is due to the completely divergent ways of application of the substances referred to by *potage*$_1$ and *potage*$_2$.

Potage$_1$, as a semisolid preparation, is recorded in the analysed material 8 times, with most of the items present in one surgical text (LSC1), cf.:

(77) (…) lewide men seyinge akynge & swellynge in a lyme þat is woundid leie þerto a **potage** [L pultes] in maner maad of eerbis & swynes greece & water & wheete flour. (Fleischhacker, a1400 *LSC1* (MS Ashm 1396), 42/12–14)
þanne bigynnen to materen þe swellynge wiþ **potage** maad of flour, oile & watir, or ellis wiþ þis maturatif (…). (Fleischhacker, a1400 *LSC1* (MS Ashm 1396), 56/4–6)
Leid aboue þe wounde a **potage** maad of.iiij parties of watir & oon partie of oile of olyue, & flour of wheete þat sufficiþ to þe medicyn, & leie þis medicyn to þe wounde (…). (Fleischhacker, a1400 *LSC1* (MS Ashm 1396), 53/2–5)

This implies that the noun was a marginal member of the lexical field of Middle English semisolid preparations.

Pultes

Following OED, the noun appeared in English writings in the 15th century with the sense 'a moist, usually heated mass of a substance with a soft, pasty consistency, applied to the skin, usually by means of a bandage or dressing, in order to promote healing, relieve pain'. This sense is a slight extension of L *pultes* 'thick pap, pottage used as poultice', from which the Middle English form was derived (OED, *poultice* n.). In the medical material, the noun is found only in surgical works (9 records), cf.:

(78) **Pultes** [L Pultes] & cathaplasma ben al oon, but propirli **pultes** ben clepid whanne þer is mele, watir, & oile wiþouten herbis. (Fleischhacker, a1400 *LSC1* (MS Ashm 1396), 331/6–8)

As the fragment above explains, *pultes,* unlike other preparations of similar consistency, contained no herbs[53].

Paste

The earliest uses of *paste* (OF *paste* and L *pasta* 'dough, pastry') in English were recorded in the late 14th century culinary writings (cf. OED, *paste* n.). Thus, originally the noun denoted (i) 'dough for the making of bread or pastry' or just (ii) 'bread or pie'. With time, *paste* started to be also used with reference to (iii) 'the dough for Communion bread' (MED, *paste* n.). This mixture of flour, liquid and other ingredients turned to make a fine composition to be applied to the skin, hence the use of the noun in 15th century medical writings with the sense (iv) 'a sealant, adhesive paste, plaster'. Only 8 instances of the noun with medical sense have been found in the analysed material, cf.:

(79) If it be in a lyme full of flesshe, þou shalt make **a past** of x partes of water and of oyle and flour of whet and ley it vpon þe postume in wounde and ley it so long ther on till all þe swellyng and Akyng be Away and þat the wounde myght whetyr. (MEMT, 1500 *LChP* (MS Wel 397), 75)
And than cautaryse hym with an hote yryn or with a brynnyng medecyne. after that lay **a past** made with the Iuse of smaleache and hony and flour of whet till it be clensyd. (MEMT, 1500 *LChP* (MS Wel 397), 88)

---

53 *Cathaplasm*, which is listed in the quotation will be discussed in chapter five devoted to the names of specifics.

Tak þe iuse of ribwort, and þe white of a neye, et ryemele, and mak a **past** and þer of a plastre, and lege vpon in a cloute (...). (MEMT, 1450–1475 *MedCh* (MS Add 34111), 132)

4.3 Solid preparations

This section discusses Middle English names for solid preparations i.e. substances that are neither fluid nor gaseous, of a dense or massive consistency and having definite shape and volume intended for both internal and external application (cf. DMD, *solid* adj. n.; OED *solid* adj.). In the analysed material 10 nouns, which could qualify for this category, have been found (cf. Table 6 below). The following types of preparations will be considered: powders (*powder, pulvis, pulver*), pills (*ball, pellet, pill, pilule, trochisk*) and suppositories (*suppository* and *pessary*). Due to the similarity in form and/or great synonymity, the nouns representing particular type of solids will be discussed together.

Tab. 6: The number of the occurrences (absolute frequencies and percentage) of nouns denoting solid preparations in the analysed material

Noun	Number of occurrences (%)	Noun	Number of occurrences (%)
ball	34 (6.6%)	powder	285 (55.4%)
pellet	40 (7.8%)	pulver	4 (0.8%)
pessary	7 (1.5%)	pulvis	15 (2.9%)
pill	10 (1.9%)	suppository	71 (13.8%)
pilule	27 (5.2%)	trochisk	21 (4.1%)

4.3.1 Powders: *powder, pulvis, pulver*

Powders, i.e. "dry, free-flowing preparations consisting of one or a mixture of finely powdered substances" (Marriott — Wilson et. al 2010: 195), were the most common solid medications used in medieval medical practice (cf. *powder* in Table 6 above). Originally, they were applied as dusting powders to dry wounds or as nose inhalations. Later, pulverised substances started to be used in the composition of ointments, pastes or liquid preparations.

The earliest English medical records, i.e. Old English writings, show that pulverized preparations were originally referred to by Gmc *dust*[54] (cf. DOE and BT, *dust* n.). In the Middle English material, this form has not been found with

54 In Old English medical writings *dust*, as a reference to a pulverized medical preparation, is recorded 101 times. According to TOE, powder was also referred to by *æmerge*,

reference to 'a pulverised substance used for medicinal purposes' as this sense was denoted by three Romance nouns: *powder*, *pulvis* and *pulver*[55].

Powder, from OF *poudre*, entered English around the 14th century with the following senses: (i) 'the mass of dry particles or granules produced by grinding, crushing or burning' and (ii) 'dust of the earth, dirt, soil' (MED, *poudre* n.; OED, *powder* n.). According to OED, in the mid-14th century the noun started to develop more specific senses, reflecting the use of a preparation for particular purposes, e.g., (iii) 'a medical substance formulated as a powder', (iv) 'a preparation used in food and cooking as a seasoning, flavouring', (v) a flammable or explosive preparation, esp. gunpowder' and (vi) 'any preparation used in alchemy or other magical practices'. The related forms of Latin origin, *pulvis* and *pulver* (L *pulvis*, *pulver-em*), whose earliest attestations were recorded in the early 15th century, were used only with the medical sense (iii), cf. also DMVE and MED, *pulver* n., *pulvis* n.

Fig. 5: The percentage of the occurrences of nouns denoting 'a medicinal powder' in the analysed material

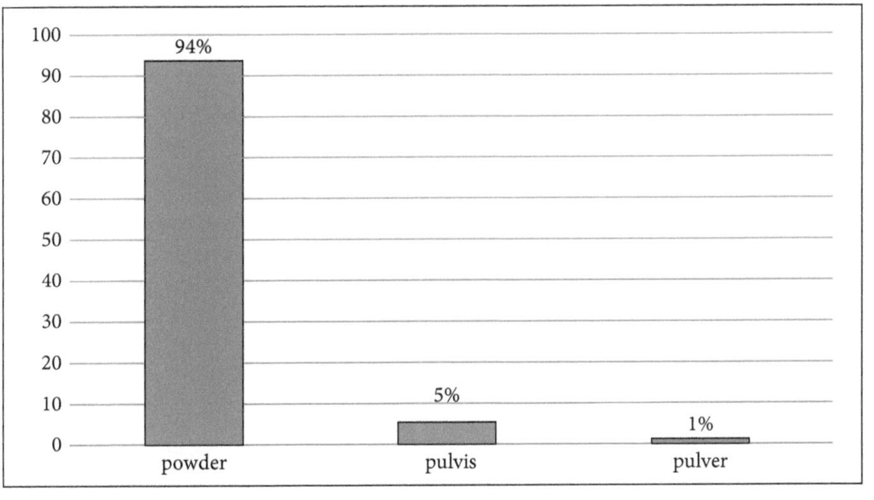

gilp, *grytt*, *myl*. These nouns have not been recorded in the examined Old English medical texts.

55 *Dust* was found only three times in complex phrases: *bark(e) dust* (2 records) and *dust of encense* (1 record). This implies that the noun was no longer used as a general term within the category of solids. Hence, it has not been included in the corpus terms analysed in this work.

As seen in Figure 5 (cf. also Table 6), out of three nouns denoting 'a medicinal powder', *powder* is the most frequent, amounting to 94% of all the powder nouns found in the medical texts. In these texts, the noun is found in the headings of recipes, usually specifying the ailment a given powder is to heal (80a), and, more frequently, within the procedure part of the recipes. Thus, the noun is often used to denote the form a given substance should take before being applied or added to another preparation (80b), cf.:

(80) a. **A pouder to do away dede flesche.** Tak saundyuere or coprose (…). (MEMT, 1440 *LDM* (MS Thornton A.5.2), 75)
A pouder þat is rede and soudes bones togyder and staunncheþ blode, is made on þis maner: Tak brisewort (…). And þis **pouder** is profitable to staunche blode and for sowdyng of þe bone and flessh. (MEMT, 1450–1475 *MedCh* (MS Add 34111), 127)
b. For nese-bledingge: Tack heschulschines a branch and bren hem and mak **puder** (bren hem) and blow þe **puder** in þe nese. (MEMT, 1330 *FCC* (MS Corp-C 388), 110)
and þan take sarcocollum and þe flour þer of and make **pouder** and do þis pouder vpon þe tent and do in þe nose. (MEMT, a1450 *CExp* (MS Add 34111), 31)

The distribution of *pulvis* and *pulver* in the analysed material (5% and 1% respectively) implies that these nouns are peripheral members of the lexical field of solids. They are used sporadically in selected surgical texts, whereas in the collection of remedy books these two forms are not recorded, unless used in Latin expressions inserted in the English text, cf.:

(81) (…) **puluis** laxatiuus. Take fyne peny wyȝt of rewbarbe, (…). (Heinrich, c1450 *HRec* (MS Add 33996), 134/20)
Puluis pro combuftionibus. Brenne in a pot þe rede nethe croppe, and þe seed þerof… (Heinrich, c1450 *HRec* (MS Add 33996), 223/3–4)

4.3.2 Pills: *ball, pellet, pill, pilule, trochisk*

Pills are small, solid dosage forms, of globular or ovoid shape. They were usually prepared by mixing medicinal herbs with honey, some juice, water or other liquid and then shaped into a form of a small ball (Marriott — Wilson et. al 2010: 27). While reading Middle English medical recipes we learn that their authors tried to be precise about the size and shape of pills. Hence, after a long list of ingredients for a pill we find statements instructing to make a pill in a shape/size of some seed(s) or fruit, e.g., nut, bean, pea, cherry, fig, cf.:

(82) And make herof **pillulis** <u>of þe quantite of a been</u>. (Getz, a1475 *GA* (MS Wel 537), 81/18–19)

(…) and þanne make **pelotys** as grete as walnotis (…) (MEMT, a1450 *ACH* (MS Roy-L 10.90), 134)

In the analysed material 5 nouns are used with reference to 'pills': *ball*, *pellet*, *pill*, *pilule*, *trochisk*. The two most frequent nouns (cf. Figure 6) in the analysed medical material are OF *pellet* (from a combination of L *pila* 'ball' and the French diminutive suffix -*ot*) and *ball* (of uncertain origin; probably from OE **beal(l*, as in *bealluc* 'testicle'; cf. DMVE, *ball* n. and MED, *bal* n.)[56]. Both terms were originally used with the sense: (i) 'a spherical or circular object'. Later, the two nouns developed more specific senses, among others (ii) 'a medicine in the form of a pill or a bolus' (MED, *bal* n. and *pelote* n.).

Fig. 6: The percentage of the occurrences of nouns denoting 'pills' in the analysed material

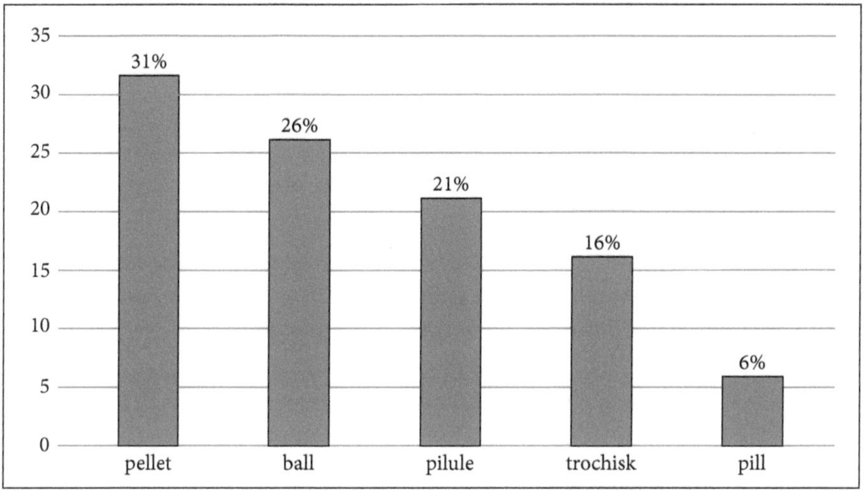

Apart from general references to medicaments in the form of pills (83a), *ball* and *pellet* are also recorded as explanatory terms for seemingly less known 'pill' terms: *pilule* and *trochisk* (83b).

(83) a. (…) make smale **pelotus** and dry hem with-outen fyer, sonne or wynd, and vse hem in this maner;(…). (MEMT, a1500 *MedW* (MSS Hrl 2378), 77)
Make of hem smale **ballis**, þat ech bal weiȝe a dragme. (Fleischhacker, a1400 *LSC1* (MS Ashm 1396), 62/4)

56 *Ball* is not recorded in Old English medical texts. According to TOE, pills were referred to by *posl* and *posling* (1 occurrence of each in Old English medical texts).

b. Ffyrst he must porge his brayn with **pelett** callyd **pillule** Iherosolimitane, wherof thus is the makyng: Take turbite, (…) and make þerof **pelatis**. (MEMT, 1474–1499 *BG* (MS Hunter V.8.6), 54)
Make þerof **pillulas** i. smale **balles**, with oximel squillitico. (MED,?c1425 *Chauliac(2)* (MS Paris angl. 25) 167/29)
Make **trociscos** (i. **pylotes**) of a noble weighte. (DMVE, a1425 *Chauliac(1)* (MS 25, Biblioteque Nationale, Paris), 165/22)

Pilule (from OF *pilule* and L *pilula*) and its shortened form *pill* appeared in Middle English medical texts at the turn of the 15th century with only one sense 'a globular medicinal solid, a pill'. *Pilule* is mostly recorded in borrowed Latin phrases, e.g., *pillule auree, pilulas cochias, pillule diacastorie*, etc. (cf. OED comment for *pilule*, cf. also Appendix B). However, in later texts, the form is also recorded as a simple lexeme denoting 'pills' in general, cf.:

(84) Distempre þou moste subtile mele of whete, with iuyse of millefoile, and make þerof **pillulez**, and giffe hym euery day in þe mornyng 3 or 4 of þam distempered with wyne. (Power, 1425 *AFS* (MS Sln 6), 60/25–26)
Pillules for to prouoke slepe: Recipe amides..croci..opii..Make þam wyth watre of roses and make **pillule** and giffe þam. (Power, 1425 *AFS* (MS Sln 6), 101/3, 5)
And let him vse þes **pillulis**: Take þe seed of melone, of gourdes, (…). (Getz, a1475 *GA* (MS Wel 537), 107/5–6)

Pill, derived from *pilule*, is recorded in much later texts, from the late 15th century (only 10 occurrences), both as a general term denoting 'pills' and in phrases specifying selected medications applied in the form of a pill, cf.:

(85) (…) he toke these pills. Re **pills** of lapis lazuli dr. j. of **pills** of hermodactillis dr. ij. misce with water of celedon & make vij **pills.** (MEMT, 15th/16th c. *TTP* (MS Sln 389), 464)
(…) medel þe poudre with þe forsayde **pille** (…). (Hallaert, a1500 *SW1* (MS Yale-M 47), 47/339–340)

The last term in the group of pill nouns, *trochisk* (from L *trochiscus*, OF *trochisque* 'small pill, lozenge'), is also a relatively late borrowing whose earliest attestations are documented in 15th century texts. In the analysed material, the noun as a single term has been encountered 21 times in only three texts (AFS, AntN, and SW2), which implies that it was still a rare term in the Middle English medical lexicon of solid preparations, cf.:

(86) Al þes grynde hem wyþ weyn and make þerof **trociscus**. (MEMT, 15th c. *AntN* (MS Ferguson 147), f. 48r)
When, forsoþ, it is cold þat it may be malaxed, enforme þerof **trocistes** vpon a table in quantite. (Power, 1425 *AFS* (MS Sln 6), 91/30)

Yeve it with **trociskys** of deliueryng of chyld that ben wreten in þe chapiter of mola matricis. (Rowland, 1450 *SW2* (MS Sln 2463), 74/2–3)

The noun is more frequent in compounds and phrases, e.g., *trochisk calidicon*, *trochisk of aldaron*, *trochisk of berberries*, *trochisk de lactea*, etc. (for more examples see Appendix B).

4.3.3 Suppositories: *suppository, pessary*

Today suppositories are usually defined as "solid unit dosage forms suitably shaped for insertion into rectum. The bases used either melt when warmed to body temperature or dissolve or disperse when in contact with mucous secretions" (Marriott — Wilson et. al 2010: 183). From Middle English medical writings we learn that suppositories were used in a broader sense than today. This medicinal preparation was inserted "into any body orifice other than mouth" (MED, *suppositorie* n.; OED, *suppository* n.), e.g., rectum (87a), vagina (87b) or even ears (87c), cf.:

(87) a. If he mai not schite oonys kyndeli in þe dai after þe quantite of mete þat he takiþ, make him a clisterie ouþer a **suppositorie** oonys ech day. (Fleischhacker, a1400 *LSC1* (MS Ashm 1396), 56/2–3)

b. A gode **suppositores** to purge wymmen. Take þe meyle of a cockle and medull yt with hony (…) and put þat in hire priuy membre, and let yt lygge þer all nyght or lenger if it nede. (Hallaert, a1500 *SW1* (MS Yale-M 47), 41/235)

c. For a man þat may noȝt wel heryn, tak þe jus of þis herbe [spurge laurel] and put it in hys erys, or ellys make a **subpositorie** of þis herbe, stamp it, and put to-gedere and ley to þe erys. (MED,?1450 *Agnus Castus* (Stockh 10.90), 176/21)

In addition, the ingredients of medieval suppositories were wound in a piece of cloth and as such applied into the body, cf.:

(88) (…) and wynde yt yn a soft lynnen cloþe and put þat in hire priuy membre. (Hallaert, a1500 *SW1* (MS Yale-M 47), 41/237–238)

(…) take tyriacull dyatessoron (…) and stampe þem to geder with coton, and make þer of a **suppositore** as gret as þy fynger and put yt in hyre pryuy membre (Hallaert, a1500 *SW1* (MS Yale-M 47), 35/161–163)

In the analysed material two nouns are used with reference to this medicinal application: *suppository* and *pessary.* Both nouns entered English around 1400 (cf. MED and OED) and are derived from the Latin forms *suppositorium* 'a medical plug' and *pessarium* 'medicated plug, especially one inserted into the vagina'. *Suppository* is a more common noun (71 records), found in all types of texts: remedy books, surgical and specialised treatises. *Pessary*, on the other hand, is much less frequent (only 7 records), and documented in treatises dealing with woman's health. This peripheral use of the noun might be explained by the fact that *pessary*, unlike *suppository*, is used with a narrower sense, i.e. 'a vaginal suppository' (89a) or, as one record of *pessary* in the analysed material reveals, a medication to cure man's genitalia (89b), cf.:

(89) a. A **pissary** to make þe moder clene (…). (Hallaert, a1500 *SW1* (MS Yale-M 47), 65/651)
(…) medel hem with cowe mylkes and gif yt hire with a **pissare** at hire priuy membre. (Hallaert, a1500 *SW1* (MS Yale-M 47), 41/255–256
Also anoþer **pissorrie** is: take jus of wormode (…); medle all these togeders & with an instrument caste it into her wombe by þe priue membre (…). (Rowland, 1450 *SW2* (MS Sln 2463), 142/33–34)
b. A mundificatif may be..a medicyn..þat is putt in bineþe (…) wiþ a **pessarie** [L pessario] for to make clene a mannes lymes wiþinne. (Fleischhacker, a1400 *LSC1* (MS Ashm 1396), 339/18–19)

4.4 Liquid preparations

This category includes terms denoting general terms for medicaments in a liquid form, i.e. preparations where at least one active ingredient is dissolved or dispersed in liquid bases (water, alcohol or oils). These pharmaceuticals are usually administered orally, but can also be introduced into other body cavities, or applied externally.

In the texts studied, 8 nouns are attested as general terms for liquid medicaments: *decoction*, *drink*, *liquor*, *oil*, *potion*, *potage$_2$*, *syrup* and *water* (cf. also Table 7). In DMVE, OED and MED all of these nouns are defined as preparations in a liquid form. The first three sections will concentrate on medicaments applied internally (*drink* and *potion*, *potage$_2$*, *syrup*), whereas the last four sections concern medicaments that were applied both internally and externally (*decoction*, *liquor*, *oil*, *water*).

Tab. 7: The number of the occurrences (absolute frequencies and percentage) of nouns denoting liquid preparations in the analysed material

Noun	Number of occurrences (%)	Noun	Number of occurrences (%)
decoction	44 (12.7%)	potion	13 (3.7%)
drink	36 (10.4%)	potage$_2$	28 (8.1%)
liquor	52 (15%)	syrup	121 (34.8%)
oil	42 (12.1%)	water	11 (3.2%)

4.4.1 *Drink* and *potion*

Two nouns are recorded to denote 'some medicinal drink': OE *drink* and OF *pocioun*. Although according to OED the earliest attestations of *drink* with the medical sense are dated back to the mid-14th century, a thorough reading of Old English medical writings has revealed that it was a common noun (107 occurrences)[57] denoting 'some medicinal drink'. In Middle English writings the noun is also documented, though much less frequently (36 occurrences). This is partly because it had to compete with other nouns which also functioned in medieval medical writings as referents to liquid vehicles carrying some medicinal ingredient. Moreover, the noun is not restricted to a medical context[58] and hence, with time, might not have been regarded as a specialised medical term. Therefore, in the 15th century texts we can observe a tendency to introduce a Romance equivalent *potion*, which, according to MED and OED, entered English with a sense related to some medical preparation, i.e. 'a liquid with healing, magical, or poisonous qualities' (MED, *pocioun* n.; OED, *potion* n.). At first, the noun still needed some explanation (cf. 90 below), which partly explains why, in contrast to *drink*, the noun is infrequent (only 13 records in the examined medical material).

(90) Ulcers of þe wombe..be couered with gode gouernaunce and wiþ conuenient **pocyon, i. drynk**, and wiþ clensynge. (MED,?c1425 *Chauliac(2)* (Paris angl. 25), 319/12)

4.4.2 *Potage*$_2$

This noun has been already discussed in section 4.2.2.4, where it is classified as a peripheral noun of the lexical field 'paste-like medicaments'. The analysed material also contains instances of the use of the noun with reference to a medicament in a liquid form (28 occurrences), often serving as a vehicle for the administration of other medicinal substances, cf.:

57 According to TOE, another noun denoting 'some medicinal drink' was *syde*, but this noun has only 1 record in Old English medical writings, in which one can also find compounds with *drink* as a head noun. These compounds specified types of medicinal drinks, e.g., *dolhdrenc* 'wound drink', *eceþ drenc* 'oximell', *miȝole drenc* 'duretic', *slǣpdrenc* 'a sleeping draught', *spiwe drenc* 'emetic', *wyrtdrenc* 'a herbal drink' etc.

58 The noun developed various senses: (i) 'a liquid swallowed for assuaging thirst', (ii) 'a beverage', (iii) 'intoxicating alcoholic beverage', (iv) 'a draught or portion of liquid'. Most of these senses were in use already in Old English (MED, *drinke* n.; OED, *drink* n.).

(91) (…) fore apostym. Take calyander & vrtyca greca & henbane (…) make poder & hete it & drynk in ale ore wyn & in **potage**. (MEMT, 15th c. *CrophB* (MS Hrl 1735), 239)
For costifnisse of wombe. Tak borage mercurie. malewis and mak **potage** þer of. (MEMT, early 15th c. *LeechB2* (MS Wel 405), 44)

4.4.3 *Syrup*

The noun developed from OF *sirop* 'sugared drink' and ultimately from Ar. *sharab* 'wine, beverage' or literally 'something drunk'. The earliest records of *syrup* in English written sources date back to the end of the 14th century with two senses: (i) 'a medicated thick sweet liquid, or a vehicle for medicines' and (ii) 'a thin sauce, usu. made from various ingredients boiled in wine used in cookery as a sweetener' (cf. MED, *sirup* n.; OED, *syrup* n.).

Syrups were very popular formulations due to high concentrations of sucrose which "prevented the decomposition of matter extracted from vegetable drugs. The syrup exerted an osmotic pressure such that the growth of bacteria, fungi and moulds was inhibited" (Marriott — Wilson et. al 2010: 29). This liquid medication was often flavoured with aromatic substances to inhibit the taste of unpleasant-tasting medicinal ingredients. A large number of records within the analysed material are compounds (*syrupus acetosus*, *syrup of violet*, *syrup of roses*, *syrup of almonds*, etc.) in which the noun *syrup* is modified by qualifying words, indicating the flavouring and/or medicinal ingredient (cf. Appendix B). As a single lexeme, *syrup* is also well represented and it is the most frequent noun of all general nouns denoting liquid preparations (121 records), cf.:

(92) **A syrup** for þys seknesse: Take þe sed of (…). (MEMT, a1475 *GAC* (MS Hunt-SM 19079), 238)
To know wedyr the morfew be curable. (…) make a **syryp** off borage and fumytere, (…) and drynke **þis syrupe** and yt scall dystroie the rote with-in-forþe; probatum est.(MEMT, c1450 *JBurg* (MS Sln 2320), 204)

4.4.4 *Decoction*

The earliest attestations of *decoction* (from OF *decoction*, L *decoction-em* 'an action of boiling down') date back to the late 14th century. The noun developed two senses: (i) 'the action of boiling in water or other liquid so as to extract the soluble parts or principles of the substance (usually animal flesh or plants/vegetables)', and (ii) 'a medicinal preparation made by boiling'. In the examined material the noun is fairly common (44 occurrences, cf. Table 7)[59] and is used to denote preparations administered both internally (93a) and externally (93b), cf.:

(93) a. In þis cas aváileþ þe myche clisteries lenitiues of watre of **decoccion** of whete brenne wiþ oyle or butter. (Power, 1425 *AFS* (MS Sln 6), 37/37)
(…) and let him swolowe doune of þe same **decoccion** into his stomake. (Getz, a1475 *GA* (MS Wel 537), 148/16–17)
b. Waische his heed with **decoccioun** of water þat þe feet & þe heed of a weþer were soden ynne. (Fleischhacker, a1400 *LSC1* (MS Ashm 1396), 61/6–7)

4.4.5 *Liquor*

Originally, *liquor* (from OF *licur, licor*) was used with the general sense (i) 'a liquid or fluid', (the first half of the 13th century; cf. OED, *liquor* n.). In the first half of the 14th century, the noun narrowed down its sense to (ii) 'fermented or distilled beverage, especially wine'. The earliest attestations of the medical sense (iii) 'a liquid preparation used in science or medicine; also, a magical potion' date back to the last decade of the 14th century (cf. MED, *licour* n.).

In the analysed material, the noun is fairly well represented (52 occurrences), denoting all three senses, cf.:

(94) a. In al maner siripis, or watres, or oþir **licour** þat gumme arabike or dragagantum shal be put yn … (Getz, a1475 *GA* (MS Wel 537), 115/10–12)
b. For ache of þe matrice. Tak an hondefulle of ditayni, (…) and a galoun of white whyne, and an half or elles als muchel of rede wyne, and stamp þes herbes forsayd in þis **licour** wiþ þe iuse of hem, (…) and drenk a litel cupfulle…(MEMT, 1450–1475 *MedCh* (MS Add 34111), 142)
c. Take whit gyngire, and rubbe hit on a wheston of norweye,(…) and wyþ þat **licoure** wasshe þe sore eye, an þat shal do awey þe perle, and saue þe eye. (Heinrich, c1450 *HRec* (MS Add 33996), 89/5–8)
Item take wermot, stamp yt and temper yt with water (…) **licore** in hys mowthe and he schall speke. (MEMT, c1450 *JBurg* (MS Sln 2320), 200)
And þan ow þe leche for to presse þe bladder with þe **liquore** atuix his honde3 and 3ette in þe **liquore**. (Power, 1425 *AFS* (MS Sln 6), 1/22–23), 77/6–8)

In (94a) the noun is used with the general sense 'liquid', whereas in the remaining sentences the noun demonstrates narrower senses. In (94b) *liquor* is clearly referring to a mixture of white and red wine, which implies that sense (ii) was also present in medical writings. This is partly due to wine being a common ingredient of various medicinal preparations, hence the use of *liquor* as an alternative

59 There are also instances of compounds with *decoction* as the head noun (cf. Appendix B).

term for a liquid mixture containing wine. Under (94c) we find *liquor* to denote a medicinal preparation, administered externally (as washing/bath) or internally (as a drink, mouth wash and/or clyster).

4.4.6 *Oil*

Oil (OE *œle*, OHG *oli*, later replaced by OF *oile, uile* 'oil' and L *oleum* 'oil, olive oil') was originally used in the sense 'unctuous liquid extracted from plants or their seeds, usually olive oil', which was a common ingredient of various medical preparations. With time (the first half of the 13th century) it started to be used with a more general sense: 'any liquid, unctuous substance' (MED, *oile* n.; DMVE, OED, *oil* n.)

Oils were very versatile substances. They were known as good cosmetics for the face, body, or hair. Also, they were used in medicine, cookery, religious practices, warfare and/or for torture (cf. MED, *oile* n.). In medical practice, oils were usually administered as anointing substances (95a) or as ingredients of ointments, pastes or other medicaments (95b), cf.:

(95) a. Þen enoynte þine hondes..wiþ **oile** of mirtilles. (MED,?a1425 **MS Htrn. 95* (MS Htrn 95), 171a/b)
b. An enplastre maad of hony..& of **oile** of violet. (Fleischhacker, a1400 *LSC1* (MS Ashm 1396), 338/28)

The frequency of *oil*, as a simple lexeme, is not very high (42 records). This, however, does not mean that the substance was not very common in medieval practice. The noun is mostly found in phrases where it is modified by qualifying words indicating the source or the main ingredient, e.g., *oil of roset, oil of violet, oil of almaundes*, etc. (cf. also Appendix B).

4.4.7 *Water*

In the analysed material only one noun (*water*) is used as a single term with reference to medicinal waters, i.e. 'liquids or solutions prepared by distillation, decoction or dissolution' (DMVE, *water* n.). Although in the medical compilations we have also records of a Romance noun (*aqua*), it is only documented in compound forms denoting various pharmaceutical waters such as *aqua ardent, aqua rosacea, aqua potabilis*, etc.[60] (cf. also DMVE, *aqua* n.). Hence, the noun is not included in the list of general terms denoting liquid preparations.

60 For more, see chapter five and Appendix B.

According to OED and MED, the noun *water* had been in common use in Old English writings, developing a variety of senses, e.g., 'one of the naturally occurring elements, i.e. air, fire, water, earth'; 'the liquid of which seas, lakes, and rivers are composed'; 'a drink, as satisfying thirst', etc. In addition, a number of uses are metaphorical, many of them of Biblical origin. As a medicinal liquid, the noun was first documented in Middle English writings with the following senses: (i) 'an herbal infusion for medicinal use, a medicinal preparation; the water in which wool has been boiled to extract lanolin; also, a lethally toxic solution, poison' (96a); (ii) 'a cosmetic lotion; toilet water' (96b); (iii) 'any of various chemical or alchemical agents' (96c), cf.:

(96) a. Lete þe wolle ligge in þe **watir** adai & anyȝt..& do þe **water** þerof into a leden vessel. (Fleischhacker, a1400 *LSC1* (MS Ashm 1396), 336/3–4)

b. A good **watir** for ladiis to makyn here face cler and fayir: Take notemuge, geryful, camamille, and a litil of confery, [etc.]. (MED,?c1450 *Stockh. PRecipes* (Sockh 10.90), 130/8)

c. The thyrde **water** of seyunte Gyle ys for to distroye many infirmiteys with in a mannys bodye, and hit ys clepid amongyste clerkes and doctoris aqua potabilis and hit ys made in this wyse. (MEMT, 15th c. *AW* (MS Hrl 2381), 29)

Although in the examined material the noun *water* as a single term is infrequent (11 records), it is much more commonly found in compounds and combinations such as *alum water*, *burning water*, *styptic water*, *water imperial*, *water of figs*, etc. (cf. also Appendix B).

4.5 Distribution of terms denoting dosage forms in three types of texts: remedy books, surgical texts and specialised treatises

As indicated in previous sections, a number of nouns used in Middle English medical compilations are characterised by a high degree of synonymity. For instance, in the group of semisolid preparations there are 11 references to salve-like preparations (*anointment*, *balm*, *grease*, *liniment*, *ointment*, *ointure*, *salve*, *uncture*, *unement*, *unguent*, *unguentum*) and 11 to paste-like forms (*electuary*, *electuarium*, *emplaster*, *emplastrum*, *entrete*, *lectuary*, *paste*, *plaster*, *potage*$_1$, *pultes*, *treat*); among solids there are at least 5 terms denoting preparations in the form of a pill (*ball*, *pellet*, *pill*, *pilule*, *trochisk*), 3 forms for a powder (*poudre*, *pulvis*, *pulver*), and in the group of liquids at least 3 nouns denote 'some medicinal drink' (*drink*, *potion*, *liquor*). Within each group we also find nouns that are similar in form, e.g., *plaster* - *emplaster* - *emplastrum*, *electuary* - *lectuary*, etc. This great variety of equivalent terms certainly made it possible to avoid repetitions. However, the analysis of their use in the texts representing different underlying traditions of medical writing (remedy books, surgical texts and specialised treatises) has shown discrepancies in their distribution. Some terms are well represented in all text-types, whereas others prevail or are typical of one type of text only.

The investigation of these writings has revealed that out of 40 nouns, 20 items have been found in all text-types (see Table 8). This suggests that they were commonly recognised terms in medical practice.

Tab. 8: The distribution of nouns (absolute frequencies) denoting dosage forms in all text-types: relative normalized frequencies (RNF per 100,000 words) are in square brackets

Noun	Remedy books	Surgical texts	Specialised treatises
ball	25 [7.0]	7 [1.8]	2 [1.8]
decoction	22 [6.2]	15 [3.9]	7 [6.2]
drink	22 [6.2]	10 [2.6]	4 [3.6]
electuary	87 [24.4]	1 [0.3]	36 [32.2]
emplaster	56 [15.7]	173 [45.1]	15 [13.4]
liquor	35 [9.8]	15 [3.9]	2 [1.8]
oil	9 [2.5]	19 [4.9]	14 [12.5]
ointment	162 [45.5]	171 [44.6]	45 [40.2]
paste	2 [0.6]	5 [1.3]	1 [0.9]
pellet	6 [1.7]	26 [6.8]	8 [7.1]
pilule	23 [6.5]	2 [0.5]	2 [1.8]
plaster	416 [116.9]	43 [11.2]	96 [85.8]
$potage_2$	14 [3.9]	5 [1.3]	9 [8.0]
potion	4 [1.1]	8 [2.1]	1 [0.9]
powder	105 [29.5]	92 [23.9]	88 [78.6]
suppository	9 [2.5]	10 [2.6]	52 [46.4]
syrup	86 [24.2]	13 [3.4]	22 [19.6]
trochisk	10 [2.8]	6 [1.6]	5 [4.5]
unguent	9 [2.5]	24 [6.2]	2 [1.8]
unguentum	1 [0.3]	7 [1.8]	1 [0.9]

In this group of nouns only one item (*ointment*) is used with a fairly equal frequency in the three types of medical writings (RNF: 45.5 in remedy books, 44.6

in surgical texts, 40.2 in specialised treatises), whereas the remaining nouns are characterised by an uneven distribution. Some of them are more common in remedy books, e.g., *ball, drink, liquor, plaster, pilule* or *syrup*, others prevail in specialised treatises, e.g., *electuary, oil, pellet, potage*$_2$, *powder, suppository* and *trochisk*, or in surgical texts, e.g., *emplaster, paste, potion, unguent* and *unguentum*. The prevalence of some terms in one group of texts reflects, to some extent, different preoccupations of physicians and surgeons. For instance, surgical works, apart from fractures or dislocations, deal mostly with healing wounds, swellings and other skin ailments, hence the use of semisolid preparations (ointments or pastes) which were usually applied externally. In specialised writings, many of which concentrate on the treatment of the intimate parts of the body, the noun *suppository* is more frequent than in other text-types.

Another group of nouns (9 out of 40 instances) consists of those found in two text-types (see Table 9 below). Most of these terms are peripheral and used occasionally. Therefore, it is difficult to explain possible reasons for the use of terms in a variety of the text. As regards some terms, their use seems to have been conditioned by the main area of interest of medical practitioners. For instance, *lectuary*, a honey-based preparation that was mostly applied orally, and an aromatic *balm* 'ointment, salve', both are typical of remedy books and specialised treatises rather than surgical texts. *Pessary* 'vaginal suppository', on the other hand, is found in specialised and surgical texts, which are mostly dealing with internal ailments.

Tab. 9: The distribution of nouns (absolute frequencies) denoting dosage forms in two text-types: relative normalized frequencies (RNF per 100,000 words) are in square brackets

Noun	Remedy books	Surgical texts	Specialised treatises
anointment	3 [0.8]	5 [1.3]	0
balm	6 [1.7]	0	1 [0.9]
entrete	23 [6.5]	4 [1.0]	0
lectuary	28 [7.9]	0	10 [8.9]
pessary	0	3 [0.8]	4 [3.6]
potage$_1$	0	7 [1.8]	1 [0.9]
salve	21 [5.9]	2 [0.5]	0
treat	10 [2.8]	6 [1.6]	0
water	8 [2.2]	3 [0.8]	0

The remaining 11 terms have been documented in only one type of medical writings (cf. Table 10). All these nouns, as discussed in the preceding sections, are marginally represented and categorised as peripheral. Therefore, it is possible that their occurrence in the texts under study is accidental and/or is a result of an individual choice of the translator. For instance, instead of using a commonly known term (e.g. *ointment*), the compiler/translator uses a less familiar noun (e.g. *liniment*). In addition, these nouns occur in only one or two writings representing a text-type. For instance, *ointure*, *pultes* and *uncture* are recorded only in the translations of the surgical writings of Lanfranc. The so-called powder-nouns, *pulvis* and *pulver*, are used in the surgical texts by Arderne and Guy de Chauliac, respectively. Similarly, *liniment* is recorded only in the translations of Guy de Chauliac's works. The noun *grease* has been found in only one collection representing remedy book tradition (HMW), while *pill* prevails in one specialised text (7 records out of 10 in TTP).

Tab. 10: The distribution of nouns (absolute frequencies) denoting dosage forms in one text-type: relative normalized frequencies (RNF per 100,000 words) are in square brackets

Noun	Remedy books	Surgical texts	Specialised texts
electuarium	0	0	1 [0.9]
emplastrum	0	1	0
grease	2 [0.6]	0	0
liniment	0	3 [0.8]	0
ointure	0	1 [0.3]	0
pill	0	0	10 [8.9]
pultes	0	9 [2.3]	0
pulver	0	4 [1.0]	0
pulvis	0	15 [3.9]	0
uncture	0	5 [1.3]	0
unement	6 [1.7]	0	0

If we look at the nouns from the etymological viewpoint, we can also observe some tendencies in their choice and distribution in the three types of medical writings.

The nouns of Germanic origin (*ball*, *drink*, *salve*, *water*) prevail in remedy books, which can be accounted for the long vernacular tradition of these medical writings. Each of these terms "had to" compete with their numerous foreign equivalents. For instance, the noun *salve* is the only Germanic word in the group of 11 salve-like preparations. And, unlike other Old English terms that are fairly well represented in all text-types, *salve* is practically restricted to the remedy books (cf. Table 9). In addition, its frequency in these texts is marginal (21 records [RNF: 5.9], cf. Table 9) when compared with OF *ointment* (162 records [RNF: 45.5], cf. Table 8). Thus, it is possible that later the noun would have been entirely removed from the medical context. This disadvantageous position of the noun in the medical lexicon of Middle English seems a bit surprising, especially that the term was the commonest salve-noun in Old English medical compilations. One possible explanation is that, as noted in section 4.2.1.3, *salve* had a wider sphere of application, being also fairly common in everyday language. Also, it might have been confused with another term, *salue* (OED, *salve* n.[5], MED, *salve* n.[2]), often used in a religious context. Thus, when looking for a term, compilers/translators of medical texts often turned to foreign terms that were less ambiguous and of a more learned and prestigious character, e.g., *ointment*, *unguent* or *unguentum*.

As regards terms of Romance origin, two nouns (*oil* and *plaster*) had already been used in Old English medical texts. Although marginally represented (24 and 4 records respectively in Old English medical texts), in time the nouns seem to have been fully assimilated in the English lexicon, which is evidenced by the data in Tables 4 and 7. In terms of frequency, *plaster* is prevalent in remedy books (RNF: 116.9), but in the other two types of writing it is also well represented. In specialised texts it is the commonest noun of all dosage terms (RNF: 85.8) and in the surgical writings it is the fourth most commonly used term (RNF: 11.2, cf. *emplaster* = RNF: 45.1, *ointment* = RNF: 44.6, *powder* = RNF: 23.9). The analysed material also shows that the noun competed with a related term, OF/L *emplaster.* Initially, *plaster* was often employed as an explanatory term for a new foreign adoption, which possibly gave *plaster* more chances to survive in the medical lexicon. *Emplaster*, a new foreign adoption, probably regarded as a more learned term for a plaster, is prevalent in the context of more learned medical texts, here surgical works (cf. *emplaster* 173 records [RNF: 45.1] and *plaster* 43 records [RNF: 11.2]), whereas *plaster* is used more often in texts representing the older tradition of medical writing (cf. *emplaster* 56 records, RNF: 15.7 and *plaster* 416 records, RNF: 116.9), see also Table 8. As regards the noun *oil*, although fairly well represented in all types of texts, its frequency, compared to *plaster*, is much lower (44 records as a simple term). The noun is much more common in compounds and phrases, cf. chapter five and Appendix B.

Other foreign adoptions also vary in their distribution. For instance, 18 terms are common to all three text-types (cf. Table 8), whereas another 18 instances have been found in either two types of texts (*anointment, balm, entrete, lectuary, pessarie, potage*$_1$, *treat*) or one type of texts (*electuarium, emplastrum, grease, pill, liniment, ointure, pultes, pulver, pulvis, uncture, unement*), cf. Tables 9 and 10. We can also observe that the distribution of these terms depended on whether they are adoptions from Old French or Latin. Most terms (29 items) which entered English from or via French are fairly well represented in all text-types. The only exceptions are *grease, pill, ointure* and *unement* that have been found in the writings representing only one text-type (cf. Table 10). In contrast, forms taken directly from Latin are mostly prevalent in learned texts. Of these, only two have been found in all three text-types (*pilule, unguentum*), whereas the remaining 5 nouns (*electuarium, emplastrum, pulver, pulvis, uncture*) are used either in the collection of surgical or specialised writings, and mostly they are restricted to one or two texts. These nouns, as observed earlier, are marginally represented and their use seems to have been the result of individual preferences of the compilers.

4.6 Summary

The general terms denoting dosage forms have been divided into three main groups: (i) semisolid preparations, (ii) solid preparations, and (iii) liquids. As a result, it is possibe to observe the rivalry between nouns that are similar in meaning and/or form but of different etymology.

The group of terms denoting semisolid dosage forms is the most numerous, with 22 instances, which have been further divided into two sub-groups: terms denoting salve-like and paste-like preparations (11 instances in each category). The former is dominated by the Romance noun *ointment*, which was introduced around the 14th century. The number of its records (378) in the examined medical material clearly shows that it outnumbers all the other nouns denoting salve-like preparations in English. As regards the group of nouns denoting paste-like mixtures, the most representative member of this group is also a noun of Romance provenance, *plaster* (555 records). Although the noun had already been present in Old English medical writings (4 records), it was at the beginning of the 14th century that *plaster* gained in importance, at least in the medical context.

In the group of solid preparations (containing altogether 10 instances) there are general terms denoting powders, pills and suppositories. In each group, at least one noun is especially dominant: *powder* (285 records), *pellet* (40 records), and *suppository* (71 records) respectively.

The last group of preparations consists of 8 general references to mixtures that were administered in the liquid form. Within this group we have nouns denoting medicinal drinks, and liquid solutions that served as vehicles for the administration of other medicinal substances and were applied either internally or externally. In terms of frequency, medicinal potions are dominated by *drink* (36 records), whereas in the latter group of terms *syrup* (121 records) is the most prominent.

Passing on to the etymology of the nouns under discussion, each group of dosage terms is dominated by the nouns that came to English either from French and via French (29 nouns), or from Latin (7 nouns). Many of these nouns are derived from the same etymological root, hence in the texts one comes across a number of variant forms for the same preparation, e.g., *electuary - electuarium*, *plaster - emplaster - emplastrum*, *unguent - unguentum*, etc. Within each group of terms denoting dosage forms, the nouns taken from French have a relatively high frequency, and are present in all text-types (remedy books, surgical texts and specialised treatises), whereas adoptions from Latin are underrepresented and often restricted to one type of text.

As regards the Germanic instances, these include one semisolid preparation (*salve*), one solid (*ball*), and two liquid forms (*drink*, *water*). Two of these nouns (*drink*, *water*) already had a medical sense in Old English writings, whereas the other two started to be incorporated in a medical context much later, i.e. in the 15th century. In Middle English medical material the nouns exhibit a low frequency of use and seem to be restricted to collections representing older tradition of medical writing, i.e. remedy books (cf. Tables 8 and 9). In addition, the nouns are often treated only as explanatory words for commonly introduced foreign forms. This, in turn, suggests that the terms of Germanic origin were not recognised as terms of a highly technical character.

In the light of the above, one can conclude that Middle English medical nomenclature was still developing. Although it is possible to distinguish a term which could be considered as a representative within each group of nouns denoting dosage forms, it seems that there was no consensus among the translators or compilers of medical works about which nouns or variant forms should be used. This is supported, partly, by the analysis of the distribution of nouns in different types of texts, which has revealed that the introduction of the term might have often depended on individual choices of the translators or compilers of medical writings.

Chapter five: Terms denoting specifics

5.1 Introduction: selection and classification

The results of the examination of Middle English medical texts have shown that, apart from general designations for pharmaceutical substances (e.g. *medicine*, *remedy*) and names of dosage forms (e.g. *ointment*, *powder*, *potion*), most terms denote medicinal preparations that could be labelled as *specifics*.

A medical *specific* is usually defined by dictionaries as 'a preparation (solid, semisolid, or liquid) intended for treating particular ailment and/or part of the body' (cf. OED *specific*, adj. n.). In the medical texts examined for this study there are many examples that fit the definition, e.g:

agrippa 'ointment for dropsy and swollen parts of the body',
diacuminum 'electuary against bloating',
diamarciaton 'ointment for stomach or breast coldness',
dwale 'a sleeping potion',
electuarium ducis 'electuary for indigestion and problems with the stomach',
nasale 'a medicinal fluid for the nose',
pilule arthetice 'a pill to purge phlegm',
rubea trociscata 'a pill/pellet for tertian fever', etc.

The context in which such terms are found allows one to identify their dosage form and the disease they are to cure.

The group of terms denoting specifics is, compared to previous groups, extremely rich in names of medical preparations and consists of at least 1646 references to about 1411 medicaments. As in previous chapters, the material has been gathered from the dictionaries and medical sources examined for the present study. For practical reasons, it has been divided into two large categories: (i) simplex terms and derivatives and (ii) compounds and phrases[61]. Within each category the names will be dealt with in sections that reflect certain semantic groups of terms. These include names indicating (i) the main ingredient(s), (ii) the origin of the preparation, (iii) part of the body, (iv) therapeutic methods, and (v) properties of the preparation. Examples that could not be included in any of the above groups will be discussed as miscellaneous names. Apart from

61 For details concerning the division of the examined terms into (i) simplex terms and derivatives and (ii) compounds and phrases see section 1.4 in chapter one.

general comments on the meaning and etymology of the terms, some space will be devoted to the discussion of the main structural patterns of the terms under discussion (e.g. affixation, pre- and/or postmodification). The last section of this chapter will concentrate on the distribution of the terms in the three types of medical texts (remedy books, surgical texts and specialised treatises).

5.2 Simplex terms and derivatives

The present section deals with 384 references to medical preparations found in the examined material. The largest group (357 instances, 93%) constitute adoptions of Latin/French names, e.g., *cicatrizative, diaborage, euperisten, mundificative, triasandal*, etc. To the remaining examples belong 21 (5.5%) forms of Germanic provenance, e.g., *breaker, chewing, fnesing, riper*, etc., 3 hybrid formations[62], e.g., *defending, frotting, straining* and 3 names of unknown origin, i.e., *colman, sorifilon, verlilium*.

The names have been divided into five semantic groups. One group contains preparations whose designations are derived from the names of the main ingredient(s). These include plant names or ingredients of animal or non-organic origin. Another category consists of names that refer to the source of the medicament, usually medical authorities. Names indicating a part of the body and a condition to be cured form the third category. The fourth group comprises terms which refer to therapeutic methods, and the fifth contains names that reflect the properties of medical preparations. There is also a group of terms whose designations do not clearly indicate the origin or the purpose of the medicament. This information is usually derived from the context or an explanation given in the text. These terms are discussed as a separate category, labelled as miscellaneous names.

5.2.1 Main ingredient(s)

Medieval pharmaceutical practice relied heavily on the use of natural substances obtained from plants, minerals or animal parts and excreta. This was in accordance with a popular view that God created the world for the benefit of man, and everything one needed, including medicines, could be found in herbs, animals or other products of Mother Nature (cf. also the line from the Book of

62 In the present study hybrid formations involve "complex forms which mix elements from the native Germanic part of the vocabulary with elements from the borrowed Romance part of the vocabulary" (Dalton-Puffer 1996: 211).

Ecclesiasticus, 38: 4: "The Lord hath created medicines out of the earth; and he that is wise will not abhor them" (kingjamesbibleonline.org). Therefore, Middle English medical writings include a large number of names for herbs, spices, stones and many other natural substances which were names for simples, i.e. medicines made of one ingredient. As regards compound medicines, which are the main focus of this study, the names of the ingredients were also the basis for naming the medicaments[63].

The examination of the dictionaries and medical writings analysed for the present study resulted in the body of material consisting of 117 instances of compound medicines[64] named after the main medical substances used in the preparation of these medicaments. All the documented instances are of Romance origin. The nouns have been divided into three groups:

(i) medicines named after the ingredient(s) of plant origin, e.g., *damaceo*, *diaborage*, *diapapaver*, etc.;
(ii) medicines named after the ingredient(s) of animal origin, e.g., *anatison*, *cantharide*, *castoreon*, etc.;
(iii) medicines named after the ingredient(s) of mineral origin, e.g., *alcofol*, *emplome*, *nutritum*, etc.

The first group is represented by 96 words, of which the most numerous are those beginning with the prefix *dia-* (79 instances), e.g., *diaborage*, *diacalamentum*, *diacapparis*, *diacarthamus*, *dianthos*, etc. The majority of the *dia-* words are names of electuaries (69 instances), whereas the remaining are names of plasters (e.g. *diaflosmus*, *diaculon*, *diapalma*, *diaquilon*), ointments (e.g. *diacroca*, *dialthe*, *dialthea*, *diamirra*), and medicaments whose dosage is not clear (e.g. *diabuglosse*, *diacison*).

The Latin prefix *dia-/dya-*[65] 'made of' (originally from Gk *δια* 'through, by') is usually combined with the nouns denoting plants or other *materia medica*, suggesting that a given herb or the like was the chief ingredient (cf. MED, *dīa-* pref.; DMLBS, *dia-* (*dya-*) pref.). For instance, the *dia-* forms listed above contained the following herbs as chief ingredients:

63 More on the difference between simple and compound medical preparations is to be found in chapter two.
64 For the full list of names see Appendix B.
65 For the discussion of ME *dia* 'a pharmaceutical preparation, a medicament', derived from prefix *dia-*, see chapter three.

borage (OF *bourache, bourage*; ML *borrago*),
calamint (OF *calamente*; ML *calamentum*),
caper (L *capparis*),
safflower or bastard saffron (ML *cartamus, -um* 'safflower'),
flowers of rosemary (ML *anthos* 'flower, rosemary'),
mullein (ML *flosmus*),
mucilages (*diaculon* and *diaquilon* < ML *chylus* 'extracted juices of plants'),
palm fruit (ML *palma* 'palm tree, palm fruit, palm branch'),
saffron (ML *crocum, crocus* 'saffron'),
marshmallows (ML *althaea*),
myrrh (ML *myrrha*),
bugloss (OF/ML *bū-glossa*) or seeds of various plants (the origin of the second element in *diacison* is unclear, probably from ML) respectively (cf. DMLBS, DMVE, MED).

The chief ingredient, indicated in the name of the medicament, is usually given as the first element in the list of ingredients used in preparing the medicament, cf.:

(97) a. **Diacaparis** is good for eueriche greuance of þe spleen and of þe lyuer, boþe newe and olde. (…) An it is þus y-made: Take of **capparis**, oz. iiii, of squille, asarum, centorie, piretre, pepir, tyme, (…). (Getz, a1475 *GA* (MS Wel 537), 239/13–24)

b. **DIACALAMENTUM**. Yt ys seyde **of calamentes**. Yt ys goode properlyche to al yuelys of þe longen of coldnes, mostwhat to hym þat beþ in alde age. (…) Take **calamynte**, ysope, blake peper, (…). (MEMT, 15th c. *AntN* (MS Ferguson 147), f. 15v)

c. **DIANTHOS**. Yt ys clepud for yt ys made **of þe floeres of þe rosemaryne**. Yt ys goode for hem þat beþe sory, slendre, þe cardyacle, þe tysyke, and yt conforteþ hem þat beþe keuerynge ou3t of heare sykenes. Take **rosmaryne**, IIII ounces; (…). (MEMT, 15th c. *AntN* (MS Ferguson 147), f. 10v)

Sometimes, as in examples (97bc), the information about the main ingredient is also given in additional comments to a recipe, here, in the initial fragments explaining the origin of the name of the medicament.

Apart from *dia-* words, there are names which start with numerical prefixes which specify the number of ingredients used in the preparation of a given medicament. *Triasandal* and *triasandri* (ML *trias* 'three' and *sandalum* 'sandalwood'; DMLBS, *triasandali* n.) denoted an electuary containing three different types of sandalwood (red, white, yellow) as the chief ingredients, cf.:

(98) **Tryasandly** [L: triasandali (B5vb)] ys good also for ptysyk & for þe stomak..& is þus ymade. Tak od saunders, boþe of þe red & þe whyte [etc.]. (DMVE, c1450 *GilbAngl(2)* (MS BL Add 30338), 72v)

Several words, being originally names of plants and herbs, extended their meaning to denote a medical preparation whose basic ingredient was a plant/herb expressed by a name. For instance, *damaceo* (ML *damascena* 'damask prunes') was one of the names for an electuary which "Ys made of plumes wyche men clepeþ damascenys." (MEMT, 15th c. *AntN* (MS Ferguson 147), f. 11r). A more common name for the same preparation was *diaprunis* (ML *diaprunis* 'made of prunes'; DMVE, *diaprunis* n.). Other electuaries named after the main ingredients are: *miclete* (ML *micleta* 'kind of herb'; DMLBS, *micleta* n.), which was used against hemorrhoids and stomach afflictions, and *pigra* (ML *picra* 'aloe; bitter purgative'; DMLBS, *picra* n.) which had purgative properties. There are also:

(i) names for ointments and plasters: *glaukin* (derived from ML *Glaucium flavium* 'poppy like plant'; DMVE, *glaukin* n.), *populeon* (OF *populeon/popilion*, ML *populeon* 'black poplar'; DMVE, *populeon*, n.), *sinapism* (ML *sinapisma*, L *sinapismus* 'plaster of mustard plant'; DMLBS, *sinapismus* n.),
(ii) names for some liquid preparations: *piment* (OF/AN *piment* 'aromatic spice'; AND, *piment* n.), i.e. a medicinal potion made by sweetening wine with honey and various spices, *ptisan/tisan* (MF/AN *ptisane*, ML *ptisana* 'peeled barley'; DMLBS, *ptisana* n.), i.e. "water þat barliche is soden yn." (Getz, a1475 *GA* (MS Wel 537), 108/2), *rose* (OF *rose*, L *rosa;* DMVE, *rose* n.) 'syrup made by boiling roses in water', *ypoquistid/ypoquistidos* (ML *ypoquistid/hypocistis;* DMLBS, *hypocistis* n.) which was a medicinal "preparation made from the thickened juice of the parasitic plant Cytinus hypocistis, which grows on the roots of the rockrose" (MED, *ipoquistidos* n.), and
(iii) names for opiates: ML *opiata*, MF/AN *opiate*, OF/AN/L *opium*, i.e. 'medical preparations containing opium poppy' (DMVE, *opiata* n. and *opium* n.).

The next group of names to consider are those that indicate the ingredients of animal origin. According to Alves — Rosa (2013: 15), whole animals, animal parts, and animal-derived products played an important role in medieval healing practices. The strong belief in the medicinal value of animal substances is confirmed by a number of works containing recipes for animal-based remedies. Also, medieval scholarly works highlighted the importance of animal *materia medica*. For instance, *De proprietatibus rerum* by Bartholomaeus Anglicuȝ (13th century; also known as Bartholomew the Englishman or Bartholomew de Glanville) contains a line stating that "nothing in a beast's body is devoid of medical value" (after MacKinney 1946 in Alves — Rosa 2013: 19).

The references to animal-based medicaments collected for the present study are less numerous than those of plant origin (15 examples). These include six instances starting with *dia-* (*diamber/diambra*, *diacastorea/diacastoreum*, *diarundines*, *diamargariton*), which shows that the prefix was not restricted to combinations with plant names. *Diamber* (ML *diambra*; *dia-* + *ambra* 'ambergris'; DMLBS, *ambra* n.[2]) was a name for an electuary containing ambergris, i.e. "waxy substance originating in intestines of sperm whale" (DMVE, *diamber* n.), *diacastoreum* (ML *diacastoreum*; *dia-* + *castoreum* 'beaver'; DMLBS, *castor/castoreum* n.) was a 'medicament derived from scent-glands of beaver' (DMVE, *diacastoreum* n.), *diarundines* (ML *diarundines*; *dia-* + *rundines* < L *hirundo* 'swallow'; DMLBS, *hirundo* n.) denoted an 'electuary containing ashes of swallows' (DMVE, *diarundines* n.), *diamargariton* (OF/AN/L *diamargariton*; *dia-* + *margariton* 'pearls'; DMLBS, *margarita* n.; AND, *margarite* n.) appeared in the sense of 'electuary containing pulverized or non-pulverized pearls' (DMVE, *diamargariton* n.).

Other instances are derivations from the nouns originally denoting animals (*anatison*, *cantharide*, *castoreolon/castoreon*) or animal products (*ceroneum*, *cerote/cerotum*, *ciroin*, *mel*). *Anatison* (L *anas*, *anatis* 'duck'; DMLBS, *anas* n.) denoted ointment containing duck's fat, *cantharide* (L *cantharis* 'blister beetle, Spanish fly'; DMLBS, *cantharis* n.) was used with reference to strong medicines made from dried cantharid beetles, *castoreolon/castoreon* were variant forms of *diacastoreum*.

The remaining names, ML *ceroneum*, ML *cerote*, OF/AN *ciroin* (all three originally meaning 'wax, beeswax'), and L/AN *mel* 'honey', are products of honey bees. The first three were names of humectants such as ointments and plasters (containing beeswax), whereas honey was a sweet medium for electuaries, syrups and healing drinks (cf. DMVE and DMLBS, *ceroneum* n., *cerotum* n., AND, *ciroine* n.[1], *mel* n.[1]).

Although medieval pharmaceutical practice was dominated by remedies of herbal and animal origin, whether simples or compounds, many physicians and pharmacists turned also to various inorganic substances (minerals, metals, clays or rocks) in the preparation of remedies. In the examined material only a few examples of compound medicines named after mineral ingredients have been recorded, e.g., *alcofol*, *alfilude*, *aurea*, *diapompholygos*, *emplome*, *nutritum*.

Alcofol, being defined as 'fine powder' (cf. MED and DMVE *alcofol* n.), is an earlier form of ML *alcohol* derived from Ar. *al-kuhul* "literally 'the kohl' – that is, powdered antimony used as a cosmetic for darkening the eyelids" (Ayto 2001: 16, *alcohol* n.). According to DMLBS *alcofol* was a 'powder used as eyesalve' (DMLBS, *alcohol* n.). Hence, in Middle English medical texts the term is recorded in the recipes for eye ailments, e.g., "A subtile **alcofol** helpyng to terez & humiditez

& relaxingez & greuoustez [*Ch.(2): grevaunces; L grauitates] of þe palpebrez."[66] (MED,?a1425 **Chauliac(1)* (MS NY 12), 127a/b).

Alfilude (ML *alfelude*) was used for treating leprosy (DMVE, *alfilude* n.). Although it is difficult to determine the main ingredient of this medicament from the sources available, MED suggests that it was a compound medicine containing steel (MED, *alfilude* n.).

Diapompholygos (ML *dia-* + *pompholyx* 'metal or dross left as deposit in furnace', DMLBS, *pompholyx* n.) was a name for an ointment containing tutty, i.e. 'crude zinc oxide'.

The remaining examples are elliptical forms for longer names of medical preparations. *Aurea* (ML *aurea* 'gold', ML *aureus* 'of gold') is used for *aurea Alexandrina*, i.e. 'a pill or bolus containing refined gold or silver', attributed to a Byzantine physician Alexander of Tralles (DMVE, *aurea* n.). *Emplome* (from Fr. *plome*, L *plumbum* 'metal lead', MED, *plum* n.) is recorded instead of *plaster of emplome*, i.e. 'a preparation including litharge'. *Nutritum* is found as a short form of *lithargyrum nutritum* 'ointment containing pulverized litharge (lead monoxide)' (DMVE, *nutritum* n.), cf. also the examples below:

(99) Balsamum ȝeue to þe pacient helpith moche. And þis passion is good **aurea** or balsamita [L: aurea alexandrina balsamita (E2vb). (DMVE, a1475 *PlatearPra* (MS Dd.10.44), 39v.)
ffor Emplome. ffor to make a **playstyr of Emplome**. Take a pynte of oyle (...). (MEMT,15th c. *WBMP* (MS Med. Misc. I), 310)
Also an oynement preued in þis caas, & is callid **Nutritum**..is þus maad: Recipe litarge of siluer, and summen taken of gold [etc.]. (DMVE, c1475(1392) *LondonSurg* (MS Wel 564), 440/2)

5.2.2 Origin of the preparation

The compilers of medical texts placed strong emphasis on indicating the source of a remedy because, as Wear (2000: 85) puts it, "much of the discourse about remedies was concerned with convincing readers that they worked"[67]. This was usually done by appealing to various medical and non-medical authorities.

The group of Middle English medical preparations named after the source of their origin comprises 12 instances. The references to the source can be

66 ME *palpebrez* stands for 'eyelids' (MED, *palpebre* n.).

67 Other ways of convincing the readers about the effectiveness of remedies involved the use of efficacy phrases (cf. Stannard 1982, Hunt 1990, Jones 1998a, Taavitsainen 2001), the use of an evaluating adjective before/after the name of the medicament (cf. Sylwanowicz 2016).

categorised into the following types: (i) medical authorities, (ii) historical figures (iii) religious and divine (i.e. God's) authority, (iv) place of origin.

The references to medical authorities involve mostly ancient physicians, e.g., Greeks: Asclepius, Hippocrates, Galen; or Arabs: Haly, Rhazes, Avicenna (Taavitsainen — Pahta 2004: 2). In the material collected for the present study, some of these authorities are found in a group of names categorised as compounds and phrases (cf. section 5.3.2). Simplex terms refer to less known physicians. For instance, *andromachi* 'pills or boluses containing pomegranate rinds, oak...' takes its name either after Andromachus the Elder who was a physician to Nero (AD 54–68) or after his son, Andromachus the Younger, who wrote a work on pharmacy (DMVE, *andromachi* n.). The next medicament, *marciaton* 'ointment for treating pains and aches' takes its name after some medical practitioner known as Martianus (cf. also: *AntN* 171: "a Martiato pertissimo medico dicitur a quo fuit inventum" after DMVE, *marciaton* n.), *mithridatum* 'antidote against poisons' is derived from a name of Mithridates[68] VI (king of Pontus in Asia Minor, 132–63 BC), whereas *philonium* 'some electuary', is attributed to a first century BC physician Philo of Tarus (DMVE, *philonium* n.).

The second group includes mostly names referring to emperors, kings or priests who either compounded a medicament or are known to have been cured with it. For instance, *adrianum*, an electuary used against headaches, migraine, eye dimness, "ys cleped of Adryan, Emperor of Rome, þe wyche yt compownde" (MEMT, 15th c. *AntN* (MS Ferguson 147), f. 2v), *iustinum*, an electuary against urinary stones and other disorders of the urinary tract, "haþe his name of Iusteyn, þe emperoer" (MEMT, 15th c. *AntN* (MS Ferguson 147), f. 27v), and *esdra*, an electuary for one feeling melancholic or for aching ears, "Ys seyde for Esdra þe prophete, yt furste compowned." (MEMT, 15th c. *AntN* (MS Ferguson 147), f. 18r). Sometimes the origin of the name is not explained in the text. For instance, *agrippa* is probably a name of an ointment said to have been used by Jewish king Herod Agrippa (DMVE, *agrippa* n.).

Appeals to religious and divine authority (i.e. God) were also a common feature in medieval medical recipes[69] since God was held as the originator of the

---

68 According to Thompson (1929: 59), Mithridates "lived in constant apprehension of being poisoned by his enemies. He endeavoured to make himself immune from their effects by taking small doses of poisonous substances daily, in combination with the antidote that he devised." According to Zebroski (2016), the medicament – *mithridatum* – contained over 70 ingredients. "The idea behind poly-pharmaceuticals was that if one ingredient did not help the patient another ingredient would." (Zebroski 2016: 55).

69 Cf. Alonso Almeida — Cabrera-Cabreu (2002) or Sylwanowicz (2017a).

virtues found in various ingredients of medicaments (plants and minerals). An example of a medicament containing in its name a reference to God is *theodoricon* (L *theos* 'God' + *dare* 'give'; DMLBS, *theos* n., *dare* v.), that is 'God-given' electuary; cf. also: "Theodoricoun of god yȝefe." (MEMT, 15th c. *AntN* (MS Ferguson 147), f. 46v). Another medicament was originally prepared with the use of 12 ingredients, hence *apostolicon* 'Apostle's plaster or ointment' (MED, *apostolicon* n.). However, as DMVE notes this name might be misleading as in "ME works the number of ingredients varies from 4 to 15" (DMVE, *apostolicon* n.)[70].

The last group of names contains nouns which inform about the place where a given medicament had been originally compounded. A fairly common term is *antioche* 'a medical preparation on the basis of wine and herbs', also found in combinations: *drink of Antioch, bewe*[71] *of Antioch, potio Antioche*, which is derived from the name of the city of Antioch (DMVE, *Antioche* n.). Similarly, *nerbon* 'black plaster' is derived from the city of Narbonne in Gascony (cf. DMVE, *Nerbon* n.; MED, *nerbone* n.). The term was coined by an English surgeon John Arderne who knew the city[72] well and as Power (1910: xiii) put it "Arderne seems to have had a soft place in his heart for Narbonne", hence the name for one of his own plasters. Interestingly, in Arderne's work we find the following explanation: "Þis emplastre is called Noirbone, for þof-al it be blak, neþerlesse it is gode" (Power, 1425 *AFS* (MS Sln 6), 91/31–32), which suggests that the term is a combination of French words *noir* 'black' and *bon* 'good' (AND, *noir* adj. and *bon* adj.). This, however, seems a whimsical comment[73] on the origin of the name for his *black plaster*.

70 An interesting account of the origins and the mysteries surrounding *apostolicon* is to be found in, for instance, Bakhtiar — Ardalan (2014).

71 ME *bewe* (from AN *bevee* 'beverage, drink'; AND, *bevee* n.[1]) is recorded only in compounds and phrases. Hence, DMVE, MED do not list it as a headword.

72 There is a fragment where Arderne talks about his patients. One of them, Adam, went to various cities, including Neyrbon, to find a specialist that might help him with fistula in ano 'anal fistula': "The forsaid sir Adam, forsoth, suffrand fistulam in ano, made for to aske counsel at all the leecheȝ and cirurgienȝ that he myȝt fynde in Gascone, at Burdeux, at Briggerac, Tolows, and Neyrbon, and Peyters, and many other places." (Power 1910: 1). For more on Arderne, see also: Zimmerman — Veith (1993) or Jones (1994).

73 Cf. also: "Narbonne had some special association for John Arderne, since he named one of his best-beloved ointments Ungt. Noirbon, adding as a pun that though it was black (Noir) it was good (bon)." (Power 1910: 108).

5.2.3 Parts of the body

This group of nouns is represented by 6 instances, all of Romance origin. The first is a name of a preparation for heart ailments, i.e. *cordial* (MF *cordial* < ML *cordialis* 'of or for the heart' < L *cor* (genitive *cordis*) 'heart'; DMLBS, *cordialis* adj., *cor* n.), derived from a MF adjective meaning 'vital, stimulating, invigorating'. In Middle English medical texts the noun form is used with the sense of 'a substance which stimulates or invigorates medicinally' (DMVE, *cordial* n., MED, *cordial* n.), cf.: "For þat þe fumez þat ar raised fro þe corrupt partie miȝt slee þe hert, be þer giffen Tiriacle to hym & oþer cordialez be ministred to hym." (MED,?a1425 **Chauliac(1)* (MS NY 12), 28a/a).

Another term, *nasale* (ML *nasale*), denoted 'a medicinal fluid for the nose' (DMVE, *nasal* n., MED, *nasale* n.). According to DMVE there is another form, *ascalle*, used with reference to the same preparation (compare examples 100ab below). However, this variant form is probably a scribal mistake influenced by ML *nascale* 'pessary' (DMVE, *ascalle* n.).

(100) a. **Nasalies** [L: nasalia (151/20)] & gargarismes & clisteries..were best whilis feuere is not þerwiþ. (DMVE, a1425 **Chauliac(2)* (Jes-C Q.G.23), 149ra)
b. Somtyme blode laste and some tyme gargarismes and **ascalles** and sternictories (i. fnesinges (…). (DMVE, a1425 *Chauliac(1)* (MS Paris angl. 25), 201/27)

Injuries of nerves and tendons could be treated with an ointment known as *nerval* (AN *nerval* < *nerf/nerves* 'nerve, tendon'; DMVE, *nerval* n., AND *nerve* n.), an ellipted form for ML *unguentum nervale*, cf.: "Take fyne aqua vite a pynte and a quarter of narvall right welle medled togeder and enoynt the place at grevyth." (DMVE, c1450 *RemLMSoc.* (MS Wel 136), 68/34).

Problems with stomach, especially indigestion or excess of humours, were solved by the application of *stomaticon* (ML/OF *stomaticon* < L *stomatichus* 'throat, stomach' < Gk στόμα = *stoma* 'mouth or mouth of the stomach'; DMLBS, *stomatichus* n., DMVE *stomaticon* n.), cf.:

(101) **Stomaticon** þat is cold is good for al vnkinde hetis of a manne stomake and quenchiþ a mannes þirste; **Stomaticon** þat is hoot is comfor[ta]ble for þe stomake and helpiþ to defie a mannes mete; And it is gode for þe greuaunce þat is in þe ouer-guttis of a mannes wombe, þer is **stomaticon** a laxatif. (Getz, a1475 *GA* (MS Wel 537), 187/18–23)

The last two terms included in this section are *sanguiboetos* (ML *sanguis* 'blood' +?boet? 'do away with'), *sanguinolent* (ML *sanguis* 'blood' + *olent* (-ulent 'full of') (cf. DMVE *sanguiboetos* n., *sanguinolent* n., DMLBS, *sanguinolens* adj.). The first was recorded as a plaster for cleansing wounds (102a), whereas the second as a styptic medicine (102b), cf.:

(102) a. I putte þerto..an emplastre þat is callyd **sanguiboetos** [L: sanguiboetos (88v)]. (DMVE, a1425 *Arderne(3)* (MS Em 69), 177r)

b. (…) wyþ farmaciez named **sanguinolent** [*Ch.(2)*: sanguinolentes, i. for bledynge woundes; L sanguinolentis]. (MED,?a1425 **Chauliac(1)* (MS NY 12), 78b/b)

5.2.4 Therapeutic methods

This group includes nouns which refer to the preparations whose names denote the way they were administered. Altogether, 12 nouns belong to this category, of which only one is of Germanic origin (*chewing*). Due to the fact that some of the names are related by meaning, they will be discussed collectively.

Three nouns, *fumigation* (MF/AN *fumigation* 'inhalation of vapours, steam bath'), *subfumigation* (OF *suffumigation*, AN *suffumigacioun* 'producing fumes'), *stuphe* (ML *stupha*, *stufa* 'hot-air, steam bath'), appeared with the sense 'fumes or vapours generated for therapeutic purposes' (cf. AND, DMLBS, DMVE, MED, OED). These were either moist or dry preparations. Thus, the fumes were either produced by boiling medicinal herbs in water or by burning them. Then, the patient's body or part of it (e.g. skin or respiratory membrane) was exposed to the fumes in order to produce a therapeutic effect (OED, *fumigation* n.), cf.:

(103) Make him a **fumigacioun** [L fumigium] to his eere wiþ hoot water, in which schal be soden maiorana & calamynte. (Fleischhacker, a1400 *LSC1* (MS Ashm 1396), 256/9–10)

Drie hem [haemorrhoids] with **fumygaciouns** [L suffumigationi]. (Fleischhacker, a1400 *LSC1* (MS Ashm 1396), 291/10)

Stufez [vr. Stuffez; *Ch.(2)*: stewes; L Stuffe] & **subfumigacions** drye & þo þingez þat prouokeþ..swet beþ helping to þis spasme. (MED,?a1425 **Chauliac(1)* (MS NY 12), 57b/b)

Apart from medicated vapours the patients were treated with 'medicated baths': *balneum* (L *balneum* 'bath'), *encatisma* (L *encathisma* 'a sitting bath'), whose preparation usually required adding medicinal herbs to hot water into which the patient was immersed (DMVE and DMLBS s.v. *balneum*, *encathisma*). The difference between *balneum* and *encatisma* lied in the fact that in the case of the latter the patient could be immersed up to the navel, cf.:

(104) **Encatisma** is seid in.ij. maners: sumtyme it is seid for a clisterie, & sumtyme for a particuler [baþ], anoon to þe nauele & non aboue þe nauel. (Fleischhacker, a1400 *LSC1* (MS Ashm 1396), 331/12–14)

What we learn from the fragment above is that *encatisma* was also used with reference to a liquid medication injected into rectum. However, more commonly used terms for this preparation were *clyster* (OF/AN *clistere*; L *clyster*) and *enema* (L *enema*), cf. also (105a). Of these two, *clyster* denoted also an instrument used for injecting enema (105b, cf. also DMVE and MED s.v. *clyster* n., *enema* n.).

(105) a. **Clisteriez** forsoþ or enema was take of a brid ynea [L ciconia] þat for akyng of his wombe toke water of þe see with his bille and kest it in to yt bihyndefurþ (…). (MED,?a1425 **Chauliac(1)* (MS NY 12), 162a/b)
b. It is brode in þe maner of an embote in þe whiche a purse of lether may be bounden, and some is with a knotte..in þe maner of **clisteres**. (MED,?a1425 **Chauliac(2)* (MS Paris angl. 25), 158a/a)

Additionally, the dictionaries (DMVE, MED) give yet another related word for a medicament injected into the sore or body cavity, *injection* (MF *injection*, L *injection-em* 'throw in'). Originally, the noun mostly denoted 'the process of pouring medicaments into wounds, etc.' (106a). With time, however, the noun was also recorded with the sense 'medicament to be injected' (106b).

(106) a. If forsoþ þu do bot litel by þe mouyng and **inieccion**, i. castyng in..cure þe wond after William minushing þe tent. (MED,?a1425 **Chauliac(1)* (MS NY 12), 76b/a)
b. Of thise thou maiste make drinke, eletuary, emplastres, vnteentes, **inieccions**, pessaria & subfumigacions. (DMVE: a1475 **GaddesRosa* (MS Sln 76),154r)

There were also medicaments applied in the mouth. *Gargarism*(a) (L *gargarisma*; DMVE, *gargarisma* n., MED, s.v. *gargarisme*) denoted 'a gargle, a medicine used to wash or rinse throat' (107a). Originally it was an echoic word that supposedly imitated the noises made while washing throat (Dirckx 1983: 25). *Mastication* (L *masticationem* 'chewing'; DMVE, *mastication* n.) and *chewing* (OE *ceowung*, DMVE *chewing* n.), on the other hand, were used with reference to any medicament that had to be chewed in the mouth (107b), cf.:

(107) a. Þou schalt make him a **gargarisme**, & þerwiþ he schal ofte waische his mouþ. (Fleischhacker, a1400 *LSC1* (MS Ashm 1396), 261/26)
b. Helpez of teþe..ar manifold..bi collucionz, i. wasshingz & gargarismez, **masticacions**, i. **chewingez**, implecionz, i. fillingez. (MED,?a1425 **Chauliac(1)* (MS NY 12), 139a/a)

The last example in the group of names denoting therapeutic methods is *frotting* (a hybrid formation containing a root from OF *froten* 'to rub, chafe' and Gmc *-ing*) which is documented with the sense 'a medicine applied by rubbing it' (DMVE, *frotting* n.), cf.:

(108) Whan any man is lette of speche for myche moysture biþ þese of whiche þou myȝt make gargarismes and **frotynges** (…). (DMVE, c1425 **BernLiliyum* (MS Ashm 1505), 123v).

5.2.5 Properties of the preparation

This section deals with the names that denote various attributes of the medicaments they refer to. There are two forms derived from colour names, e.g., *blanca* and *rubea*. The preparation known as *blanca* (ML 'white') had its name from the humour it purged: "Yt ys clepud for yt purget whyte humores, þat ys to sey, flewmetyke humores." (MEMT, 15th c. *AntN* (MS Ferguson 147), f. 7r), whereas *rubea* (L *rubeus* 'red'), probably short for *rubea trociscata* 'red pills or boluses containing spices; used against fevers' (DMVE, *rubea trociscata* n.), denoted the colour of the medicament: "Yt ys clepudde rubea, for yt ys rede of colour;" (MEMT, 15th c. *AntN* (MS Ferguson 147), f. 40r). Another name, *benedicta* 'electuary containing purgative drugs' (DMVE, *benedicta* n.), puts emphasis on the fact that a preparation is exceptional as it guarantees blessing, cf.: "Yt ys clepud for alle men þat ys reseyued yt ys yblessed." (MEMT, 15th c. *AntN* (MS Ferguson 147), f. 7v). Yet another term, *local* (L *localis*; MED, *local* n.), indicated topical medications, i.e. those applied locally. The largest group of names are those which describe "drugs' actions", i.e. ways of remedying various conditions; healing properties of medicaments. An examination of the dictionaries and medieval medical writings has shown that this group of names of medicines was extremely rich in terms, with 190 instances identified and collected. Many of these are related by meaning, and this, obviously, called for grouping them into categories.

A starting point was to classify them, at least partially, according to the principles of the humoral theory[74]. The task of a physician was to restore the humoral balance by prescribing medicaments that would counterbalance the excess of one of the humours. For instance, from many recipes we learn that a pain in the eyes, being the result of the excess of hot humours, should be treated by applying *mitigatives* 'preparations alleviating pain' and/or *repercussives* 'preparations drawing back morbid matter', both being cold medicaments. This suggests that the nouns under discussion could be divided into four main groups, i.e. hot, cold, dry and moist medications.

However, many terms were characterised by two, often contradicting, qualities. For instance, there were two types of *corrosives* 'preparations consuming morbid matter': moist and dry, cf.:

(109) And in drye yȝen, vse **moyste corosi/ues**; and in moyste yȝen, **drye corosiues**; (…). (Getz, a1475 *GA* (MS Wel 537), 53/21–22)

74 The principles of humoral theory are discussed in more detail in chapter two.

As regards some terms it was difficult to determine the quality of the medicament as the authors/compilers of medical texts often failed to provide such information. In addition, no single text offers a comprehensive description of all preparations and their qualities. Even if there happened to be some passage devoted to these terms, the focus was only on selected names. For instance, in the last section of Lanfranc's *Science of Cirurgie*, the author discusses the following categories of medicaments: repercussives, resolutives, maturatives, mundificatives, regeneratives and consolidatives, cauterisatives and corrosives, mollificatives and softening. This list is limited to the medicaments that he "lernede hem of wise doctouris & of philosophoris, & alle þei ben aproued" and that were suitable for surgical treatment. Lanfranc explains lack of other instances of medicaments as follows: "…þere is no man þat can telle alle þe noumbre of medicyns but oonli god." (Fleischhacker, a1400 *LSC1* (MS Ashm 1396), 328/ 14–15, 12).

Taking into account the above complexities, it was necessary to verify the meaning of each collected noun in order to create groups of terms sharing the same sense. For instance, terms denoting 'medicines causing body tissues tighten/narrow' have been included in a group of closing medicines. Another step was to examine their use in the context. This allowed to observe that some terms with a seemingly overlapping form (cf. *mordificative* 'strong purging medicine' and *mortificative* 'medicine burning and destroying bodily tissue') or sense (cf. *conglutinative* 'closing medicine, causing body tissues to tighten' and *consolidative* 'closing medicine, promoting tissue growth') had to be excluded from one group and put into another. Sometimes a separate category had to be created. As a result, the collected words have been divided into the following nineteen groups:

(i) nouns denoting closing medicines, which are further subdivided into two types:
  (a) astringent medicines "þat makiþ þe lippis of a wounde soude togidere" (Fleischhacker, a1400 *LSC1* (MS Ashm 1396), 344/30), i.e. 'causing body tissues (e.g. skin) to tighten': *aggregative, closer, conglutinative, conglutinativum, consouder, indurative, souder*;
  (b) cicatrizant medicines "þat makiþ hard fleisch to arise in þe stide of skyn" (Fleischhacker, a1400 *LSC1* (MS Ashm 1396), 344/32–33), 'i.e. promoting tissue growth': *cicatrizative, consolidative, generative, incarnative, regenerative, sigillative, solidative*;

(ii) nouns denoting constricting medicines that "staunche þa flowing of þe humour" (Getz, a1475 *GA* (MS Wel 537), 93/12), i.e. 'narrowing, contracting, staunching': *constrainative, constrictive, constrictory, restrictive, stypter, styptic, styptica, strictory, thinner*;

(iii) nouns denoting opening medicines that “open pores in mannes bodi þat ben y-stoppid” (Getz, a1475 *GA* (MS Wel 537), 218/10–11), i.e. ‘promoting dilation or opening of e.g., body pores’: *aperitiva, aperitive, diaphoretic, dilative, leptomer, liptomer*;

(iv) nouns denoting cleansing medicines “þat doiþ awei hore in woundis & superfluite” (Fleischhacker, a1400 *LSC1* (MS Ashm 1396), 339/15–16), i.e. ‘having the quality of cleansing, scouring, or washing away impurities; used externally’: *ablution, abstersive, cleanser, lavament, lavatory, mundificative, mundifier, saramitum, washer, washing*;

(v) nouns denoting purging medicines “þe whiche þrowen oute þe mater” (DMVE, a1425 *Chauliac(1)* (MS Paris angl. 25), 586/5), i.e. ‘purging excess of morbid humours through, e.g., laxation, perspiration, vomiting’: *attractive, catharticum, cholagogue, deoppilative, digestion, digestive, diuretic, diuretica, drawer, eductive, evacuative, evaporative, expressure, expulsive, extractive, fleumagogue (fleumagogon, fleumagogum), fnesing, (h)iera, laxative, melagogue, mordificative, pharmacy, purgacia, purgation, purgative, sternutory, sudatorium, tractative, trifera, urinative, vaporative, vomit*;

(vi) nouns denoting repercussive medicines “þat repellen or driuen aȝen þe mater” (DMVE, a1425 **Chauliac(2)* (Jes-C Q.G.23), 66ra), i.e. ‘drawing back, repelling morbid matter’: *apocrustica, blisterer, consumentia, consumptive, impulsive, (re)percussive, rebounder, repercussion, repercussive, repercussivum, repulsive, restrainer, stupefactive, treacle, waster*;

(vii) nouns denoting corrosive medicines “þat bursteþ or brekeþ and brenneþ þe skyn and þe flesche” (DMVE, a1425 *Chauliac(1)* (MS Paris angl. 25), 445/5–6), i.e. ‘destroying and/or burning bodily tissue’: *aldaron, breaker, capitel, capitellum, caustic, cauterisative, corrosive, corsie, fretter, martencium, mordicative, mortificative, putrefactive, ruptory, ulcerative*;

(viii) nouns denoting dissolving medicines “þat mowen dissolue þe mater of þe sekenes riȝt as þe hete of þe sunne dissolueþ yis or snowe into watir” (Getz, a1475 *GA* (MS Wel 537), 36/15–16), i.e. ‘melting, dissolving or breaking up morbid matter’: *colliquatif, dissolutifice, dissolutive, dissolventia, incisiva, inscisive, resolutive*;

(ix) nouns denoting reducing medicines “þat maken þe mater sotil” (Getz, a1475 *GA* (MS Wel 537), 137/13), i.e. ‘thinning humours, vapours, secretions’: *attenuancia, extenuative, rarestiva, rarifactive, subtiliative*;

(x) nouns denoting drying medicines “þat dryen & wasten þe mater” (DMVE, a1475 *PlatearPra* (MS Dd.10.44), 18v), i.e. ‘increasing the dry quality in patient’s body’: *dessicantia, dessicative, dryer, exsiccative, siccative*;

(xi) nouns denoting "medicin for to make moyste" (DMVE, a1475 *PlatearPra* (MS Dd.10.44), 94r), i.e. 'increasing the moist quality in patient's body': *humectantia, moister*;

(xii) nouns denoting suppurative medicines that "make þe postem ripe" (Getz, a1475 *GA* (MS Wel 537), 229/18), i.e. 'promoting formation of pus': *maturativa, maturative, riper, suppurative*;

(xiii) nouns denoting palliative medicines that "comforte þe membre þat akiþ" (Getz, a1475 *GA* (MS Wel 537), 36/20–21), i.e. 'soothing and/or alleviating pain': *abater, anodyna, assuager, comfortative, comforter, dwale, mitigative, narcotic, narcoticum, relaxative, requies, sedative, soporative, swager*;

(xiv) nouns denoting mollifying medicines "þat nesshe þat is hardid (…) þat smoþe þat was roughe, and sharpe, and harde, þorouȝ drynes" (Getz, a1475 *GA* (MS Wel 537), 108/21–22), i.e. 'with softening effect': *bath, epithema, epithemation, foment, fomentation, lenificative, lenitive, lesser, molliative, mollificative, mollifier, mollitive, remollitive, softener, softer, suppler*;

(xv) nouns denoting "hetynge medecynes" (DMVE, a1425 *Chauliac(1)* (MS Paris angl. 25), 326/26), i.e. 'increasing body heat': *calefaciencia, calefaction, calefactive, calefactory, chafer*;

(xvi) nouns denoting "colynge medicynes" (MED,?a1425 **Chauliac(1)* (MS NY 12), 27a/b), i.e.: 'reducing body heat': *enfreider, extinguentia, frigidative, infreider, infrigidative, keeler, refrigerative*;

(xvii) nouns denoting preventive medicines that "defendiþ a membre fro corupcion" (Fleischhacker, a1450 *LSC2* (MS Add 12056), 82/26), i.e. 'maintaining health and protecting from, e.g. infection': *conditum, conservative, defender, defending, defensive, preservative, refrainer, refrenative*;

(xviii) nouns denoting restorative medicines "for man or womman þat is consumed in sijknes to restore hem in hasty tyme" (DMVE, *RemSl.* (MS Sln 73a), 122v), i.e. 'restoring, improving health; strengthening': *acutives, fastener, illuminative, restaurative, restorative, resumptive, sanative*;

(xix) names denoting "alteratiuis.i. of chounchynge medicins" (DMVE, a1475 *PlatearPra* (MS Dd.10.44), 22v), i.e. 'medicines changing quality, e.g. from hot to cold': *alterative, alterer.*

Additionally, there are five nouns whose names reveal healing properties, but they do not fit in any of the above categories: *knittere* 'a medicine causing bones to mend', *leader* 'a preparation that conveyed curative substances', *preparative* 'a medicine given before treatment or other medicines', *provoker* 'medicine promoting discharge of urine', and *straining* 'a filtrated concoction' (cf. DMVE, MED).

Etymologically, the nouns can be divided into three groups. The first, and the least represented, is a group of hybrid formations which includes 2 combinations of French roots and Gmc *-ing*, e.g., *defending* (OF *defendre* 'protect, defend'; MED, *defenden* n.) and *straining* (OF *estreign* 'bind, fasten'; MED, *streinen* v.). The second group includes 19 words of Germanic origin (*bath, breaker, cleanser, dwale, dryer, drawer, fastener, fnesing, fretter, keeler, knittere, leader, lesser, riper, softener, softer, thinner, washer, washing*). Most of the nouns are formations of a verb combined with the suffix *-er* (15 items). A thorough reading of Middle English medical writings has revealed that native words were, in most cases, used as explanatory terms for the names of foreign origin, cf.:

(110) Cap. iiij of **Mundificatiuis**, þat beþ **clanseres**. (Fleischhacker, a1450 *LSC2* (MS Add 12056), 6/8)
Of tooþ þat is loos & feble..Ðei ben holpen wiþ **resumptifs** or **fastners**. (DMVE, a1425 **Chauliac(2)* (Jes-C Q.G.23), 322rb)
Cap. iij of **Maturatiuis**, þat buþ **Ripers**. (Fleischhacker, a1450 *LSC2* (MS Add 12056), 6/7)
If þe wombe be constipat (...) let ministre to him som **lenitif.i. softer** of þe wombe. (DMVE, a1425 **Chauliac(2)* (Jes-C Q.G.23), 245ra.)

The third and the largest group contains 169 names of Latin or French origin. The majority of these nouns (107 items, 63%) are derivatives ending with the suffixes *-ive* and *-er*: 82 items (48%) and 25 items (15%) respectively, both being used to form agent nouns. The suffix *-ive* has its origins in L *-īvus*, meaning 'having the quality of, or tending to an action', which was added to verbs to form adjectives, e.g., *attractīvus, curatīvus, dīgestīvus*. The earliest *-ive* records in English, dating back to the turn of the 14th century, were Anglo-Norman loans, originally ending with *-if*, fem. *-ive* (cf. OED, *-ive* suf.; Miller 2006: 203–205, Kaunisto 2009: 75). The change into *-ive*, as Marchand (1969: 315) states, was "partly due to the influence of Latin, partly a result of the place of the main stress". Although *-ive* was originally an adjectival suffix, many of these adjectives, already in Latin, were used as nouns denoting 'agents or things that performed some action' (OED, *-ive* suf.; MED *-ĭf, -īve* suf.). Hence the presence of at least 82 names for medicaments that were derived from adjective forms ending with *-ive* in Middle English medical writings.

In case of *-er* forms it is often difficult to determine whether these are combinations of verbs of Romance origin with the Middle English suffix *-er* (< OE *-ere*) or adoptions from French. This is partly because in Middle English "there was frequent contamination between E *-er* and the French forms", in particular French agent nouns in *-(i)er(e)* (Miller 2006: 142). At least 16 out of 25 collected nouns, according to DMVE, MED and OED, are combinations of a Middle

English verb and the suffix *-er*, e.g.: *abater* (*abate* 'to relieve, mitigate' < (OF *abatre*) + *-er*), *blisterer* (*blister* 'to cause blistering' < (OF n. *blestre*) + *-er*), *moister* (*moist* 'to give the quality of moistness to the body' < (OF *moistir*) + *-er*), etc.

The remaining nine nouns (*chafer, closer, comforter, defender, enfreider, infreider, leptomer, souder, waster*), according to the same dictionaries, seem to have been adoptions of Romance forms, e.g., *comforter* < OF *conforteur*, AN *confortere*, *defender* < OF *defendeor*, MF *defendeur*, AN *defendour*, *infreider* < OF *enfroidir*, AN *enfreidir*, etc. However, two of these eight nouns, *chafer* and *waster*, are often explained as either combinations of ME *chaufe* 'to warm, heat' and *waste* 'to consume' with ME *-er*, or adoptions of MF *chauffoire*, AN *chaufour* (DMVE s.v. *chafer*) and AN *wastur* (DMVE s.v. *waster*), respectively.

Other examples consist of forms that can be divided into the following five groups:

(i) adoptions of Latin plural nominative/accusative present participles and/or adjectives used as substantives, characterised by the neuter ending *-a*, e.g., *anodyna, aperitiva, apocrustica, attenuancia, benedicta, blanca, calefaciencia, consumentia, desiccantia, dissolventia, diuretica, extinguentia, humectantia, incisiva, maturativa, purgancia, rarestiva, rubea, styptica*;

(ii) adoptions of Latin nouns in nominative *-um* forms, e.g.,[75] *capitellum, catharticum, conditum, conglutinativum, martencium, narcoticum, repercussivum, saramitum, sudatorium*;

(iii) nouns with *-ory*, a suffix originally forming nouns denoting "things" used in some process. This suffix has its origins in Fr. *-orie* (hence in Middle English texts most words were recorded with variant forms *-orie, -orye*) and was a form for the adaptation of Latin neuter nouns in *-orium* and adjectives in *-orius* (cf. OED, *-ory* suf.; Marchand 1969: 336), e.g., *calefactory* (< L *calefactorius*, ML *calefactorium*), *constrictory* (< L *constrictorium*), *lavatory* (< L *lavatorium*), *ruptory* (< L *ruptorium*), *sternutory* (< L *sternutatorius*), *strictory* (< L *strictorium*);

(iv) nouns with *-ion*, a suffix of Romance origin forming nouns of condition or action (OED s.v. *-ion*; cf. also *-tion, -ation*). The collected examples are direct loans from French or Latin, e.g., *ablution* (< OF *ablution*, L *ablutionem*), *calefaction* (< OF *calefaction*, L *calefaction-em*), *digestion* (< OF *digestion*, L *digestion-em*), *epithemation* (< Fr. *epithimation*), *fomentation* (< MF/AN

75 For the discussion of "English" *-um* forms see chapter one, section 1.4 (Guy de Chauliac's comment on nominative *-um* forms).

fomentation, < L *fomentation-em*), *purgation* (< OF *purgacion*, L *purgatio*), *repercussion* (< OF *repercussion*, L *repercussio*);

(v) nouns with *-ic*, a suffix representing MF *-ique* and L *-ic-us*, primarily forming adjectives (OED, *-ic* suf.). Many of the adjectives were also used as substantives. The collected examples include: *caustic*, *diaphoretic*, *diuretic*, *narcotic*, *styptic*.

There are also nouns that do not belong to any of the above discussed groups. The examples include, among others:

(i) *corsie*, a reduced form of *corrosive* (DMVE and OED s.v. *corsie*),

(ii) *dissolutifice* containing suffix *-fic* that was attached to verbal stems in the sense 'causing to' (DMVE s.v. *dissolutifice*; OED *-fic*, suf.), and

(iii) direct loans from French or Latin: *capitel* (< Fr. *capitel*; DMVE s.v. *capitel*), *epithema* (< L *epithema*; DMVE, *epithema* n.), *(ex)pressure* (< Fr. *pressure* and/or L *pressura*; DMVE s.v. *pressure*; MED s.v. *expressure*), *foment* (< Fr. *foment*), *lavament* (< L *lavamentum*; DMVE s.v. *lavament*), *pharmacy* (< OF *farmacie* and/or L *pharmacia*; DMVE, *pharmacy* n.), *requies* (< L *requies*; DMVE, *requies* n.), *vomit* (< OF/AN *vomit*, L *vomitus*; DMVE, *vomit* n.).

5.2.6 Miscellaneous names

This section concentrates on the names of medical preparations that do not fit in with any of the groups discussed earlier. This group of nouns comprises 42 items of Romance origin and Gmc *mead*. There are several reasons why these names are discussed separately. Firstly, most of them are not "transparent", e.g., *diaprunis*, *diacastoreon*, *cantharide*, etc., where the main ingredient is part of the name of the medicament, or *defensive*, *maturative*, *purgative*, *strictory*, etc., where the healing property is explicitly denoted by the name. Secondly, some words, if encountered by an inexperienced practitioner, might have been misinterpreted due to their ambiguity. And, last but not least, some words are not very common or are restricted to only one type of medical context (e.g. in recipes for eyes).

Let us start the discussion with the medicaments whose names might have been, to some extent, deceptive, e.g., *basilicon*, *stephannia*, *tryufiloun*.

The form *basilicon*, according to MED, was used with two senses: (i) 'a garden herb of the mint family, basil' (MED, *basilicon* n.[1]) and (ii) 'an ointment' (MED, *basilicon* n.[2]). The second sense is also recorded in OED and DMVE.

Stephannia, although not documented in DMVE, MED or OED, is recorded in one collection of Middle English recipes as the name of a compound medicine "for ache of þe syde, to hym þat soffreþ flux of blode, aboueforþ or beneforþ,

(...)" (MEMT, 15th c. *AntN* (MS Ferguson 147), f. 42r). It is possible that the name is derived from ML *stephanina* 'a plant with medicinal properties, perh. liverwort' (DMLBS, *stephanina* n.).

Tryufiloun is recorded only in *Antidotarium Nicholai* (AntN), as a remedy "for hym þat haueþ þe quarteyn, and þe cotidian." (MEMT, 15th c. *AntN* (MS Ferguson 147), f. 46r), i.e. for two types of fevers: quartan, with attacks every third day, and quotidian, with daily attacks (cf. DMVE s.v. *quartan* and *quotidian*). In MED and OED the noun is documented only with the sense 'a plant with triple or trifoliate leaves' (*trefoil* n.).

Thus, *basilicon, stephannia* and *tryufiloun*, were the names of both, medicinal plants/herbs and compound medicaments. It would be then expected that the recipes for compound medicines named after these three terms should list, among other ingredients, the names of plants/herbs to which these names refer to, i.e. basil, liverwort, and clover. However, a thorough reading of the recipes has revealed that none of these plants/herbs was used to prepare these medicaments.

Another group consists of such terms as *alcalcolon, antamaron, aragon, athanasia, diacomeron, philantropos,* all of which might also have been puzzling as, at first sight, their reference to pharmaceuticals is not that apparent and they, surely, required some explanation. In the material examined for the present study, all the above names, except for *aragon* (also found in the combination as *unguentum aragon*), are recorded in the collection of recipes known as *Antidotarium Nicholai*. A characteristic feature of this collection is that its compiler starts the recipes with a brief account on the origin of the name of the medicament and/or an explanation of its meaning. The following explanations are given for the names listed above, cf. MEMT, 15th c. *AntN* (MS Ferguson 147):

(111) **alcalcolon** "þat ys to sei a goode bygynynge." (f. 4v),
antamaron "That ys to sey a3eyn deþ." (f. 5v),
athanasia "That ys to sey no3t dedlyche." (f. 4r),
diacomeron "þat ys to sei, bryngyng a man fram deþ to lyue." (f. 9v),
philantropos "Yt ys to vndurstondynge mannys frende." (f. 25v).

As regards *aragon* 'ointment cointaining animal fats, beeswax, gums, laurel-berry oil, herbs', DMVE provides the following quotation from the Latin version of *Antidotarium Nicholai*: "aragon id est adiutorium.", where *adiutorium* means 'help, assistance' (DMLBS, *adiutorium* n.). What we learn from all these explanations is that some of the medicaments have promising virtues, e.g., they can prolong our life (*antamaron, athanasia, diacomeron*), guarantee relief (*alkalkolon, aragon*), or can be regarded as a man's friend (*philantropos*). However, their peculiar definitions are not very illuminating and sometimes one has to go through the whole recipe to find out what ailments these medicaments were meant for.

Similarly, *acaristum*, *combrota*, *euperisten*, *litontripon*, *opopira* required some explanation, cf.:

(112) **acaristum**: Wyþouȝt nombur yt ys vndurstonde. Yt ys goode for strytenes of þe breste, þe wyche comethe of þe coldenes; yt ys goode for hem þat beþe asmatic and arteriatic, and to hem þat cowgheþ, and to hem þat haueþ the flyx of þe flewme. (MEMT, 15th c. *AntN* (MS Ferguson 147), f. 3v)
combrota: Combrota [L: combrota (83v)], þat is to seye a medicine þat is schedynge or sokynge inward (DMVE, a1425 *Arderne(3)* (MS Em 69), 167r)
euperisten: And ȝif þat it beo so þat þe man þat haþe þis sekenes and haþe þe wombe yswole be long tyme do ȝif þe seek ieralagodion or elles theodoricon or elles euperisten and enoynt in bare welle wiþe diamarciaton or elles wiþ aragon (MEMT, a1450 *CExp* (MS Add 34111), 43)
litontripon: þurlynge þe ston yt ys vndurstonde. Properlyche yt brekeþ þe stone and putyþ hym ouȝt, ȝef yt be on þe reynes or on þe bleddre. (MEMT, 15th c. *AntN* (MS Ferguson 147), f. 28v)
opopira: Yt ys seyde of jois of fuyre. Opos on greke ys yois on latyn. Pir, þat ys to sey, fuyre on englyche; where þoroȝ opopira, þat ys, yois yfuyrede or elles ysete a fuyre. (…) yt heleþ þe palsye of þe tunge, and of þe yȝen, þe mowþe, and of þe þrote, þe hande, and of þe feet. (MEMT, 15th c. *AntN* (MS Ferguson 147), f. 33r)

Out of the five names, only *euperisten* is not explicitly defined. In the material examined for the present study the quotation above is the only fragment where the term has been recorded. The noun is not defined by MED and DMVE, though from the fragment above we can learn that it must have been the name of some medicament, probably a purgative electuary. The noun is listed as one of the alternative preparations, together with *ieralogodion* and *theodoricon*, both being names of purgative electuaries (cf. MED, *jeralogodion* n. and *theodoricon* n.). As for the remaining four terms, we can find remarks on the ailments they cure and even some etymological information (cf. *opopira*).

As already noted in sections 5.2.1 and 5.2.2, there is a group of compound medicaments, whose names pointed out the number of ingredients a given preparation is composed of (cf. the discussion of *triasandal*, *triasandri* and *apostolicon*). To this group of names we can add: *climax*, *(dia)catholicon*, *diatesseroun*, *triapharmacum* and *tetrapharmaca*. According to DMVE, *climax* 'an electuary containing sixty herbs' was derived from ML *climax Hermetis* 'ladder of Hermes'. It is probably "so called because the 60 herbs were added to the mixture in groups of four, with the amount taken increased each time." (DMVE, *climax* n.). Similarly, *(dia)catholicon* 'an electuary or salve for general use', was called so because of its manifold composition (OED, *diacatholicon* n.). However, in the case of this medicament the exact number of ingredients is not specified. The last three names, though including significantly fewer ingredients, seem to be more precise. *Diatesseroun* (< ML *tessara* < Gk 'four'; DMLBS, *tessara*) "is made of four thyngys, þat is to sey of myrre, arystologye id est galyngale round, gencyan and bayes of laureres." (DMVE, c1475 *TrotSecreta* (MS Jes-C Q.D.1), 71v). Likewise, *triapharmacum* and *tetrapharmaca*, being combinations with ML numerical prefixes *tria-* < Gk 'three' and *tetra-* < Gk 'four', denoted the exact number of ingredients used in the preparation of ML *pharmacum* 'drug, medicine' (DMLBS, *pharmacum* n.), cf.:

(113) **Triafarmacum** [L triafarmacum]..is made de farina frumenti, i. mele of whete, aqua, & oleo cocte to-gider; (...). (Wallner, 1425 *GCA1* (MS NY 12), 2.43/13)
Tetrafarmaton[76]..is ycompounnede of oile, piche, wax and schepis talowe. (DMVE, c1450 *Theodoric(1)* (MS Pep 1661), 182)

The above list of "numerical" names can be supplemented with *qvadrineroun* (< ML *quattuor* 'four', DMLBS, *quattuor*), probably an electuary that "haþe his name of IIII þingis. Yt ys goode for hym þat bethe asmatyke and to hym þat haueþ þe cowghe yclepud catarrus. Yt ys goode also for ache of þe stomak of coldnes; yt procureþ digestioun, yt releueþ feble reynes." (MEMT, 15th c. *AntN* (MS Ferguson 147), f. 39v). Unlike the previous examples, this name emphasises the number of uses of a preparation.

The next list of names of medicaments includes words for liquid and semisolid specifics. The first group is represented by:

claret (OF *claret* 'clear, light coloured, e.g. wine' < L *clarus* 'clear'; MED, *claret* adj.), i.e. a drink based on wine, honey and medicinal herbs (MED, claret n.[1]);
colature (MF/AN *colature* 'filtrated, strained liquid'; DMVE, *colature* n., DMLBS, *colatura* n.), i.e. some medicinal concoction;
julep (OF *julep,* ML *julab* 'rose water'; DMVE and MED, *julep* n., DMLBS, *julab* n.) denoting 'a medicinal syrup made of sugar and water and used by itself or with other ingredients';
lycium (L *lycium* 'juice or sap of a thorn-bush') 'juice extracted from various plants' which was often powdered before application (DMLBS and DMVE, *lycium* n.);
mead (OE *medu, meodu*) 'a medicinal potion prepared by fermenting honey with water' (DMVE, *mead* n.),

76 *Tetrafarmaton* is an alternative form for *tetrapharmaca* (cf. DMVE, *tetrapharmaca* n.).

ordeatum (ML *ordeatum/hordeatus* 'made of barley'; DMLBS, *hordeatus* n.) 'a drink made by boiling water and crushed barley';
sape (L *sapa* 'new wine boiled thick'; OED, *sapa* n.) which was a medicinal concoction based on sweet wine (DMVE, *sape* n.), cf. also:

(114) Make þerof [various spices] a powdre, & wiþ two pound of hony and wiþ þre potelles [of wine] make þerof a **clarete** [L claretum]. (MED,?a1425 **Chauliac(2)* (MS Paris angl. 25), 189a/b)
Þe **colature** i. þe streyned mater. (MED,?a1425 **Chauliac(2)* (MS Paris angl. 25), 112b/a)
Julep - þat is a sirup maad oonly of water & of sugre. (Fleischhacker, a1400 *LSC1* (MS Ashm 1396), 76/9)
Licium is made þus: Take þe leueȝ of caprifoile and brisse þam in a morter, and þriste out þe iuse, and putte in a brasen vessel or of glasse, and drie it at þe sunne (…). (Power, 1425 *AFS* (MS Sln 6), 44/30–33)
When she schal slepen ȝif here to drynk a drynk þat is callede in phisik mellicratum, in oþer facultes meldo or medo, anglice **mede**. (DMVE, c1450 **DanielUric* (MS Roy 17.D.1), 106 rb)
It suffiseþ to hym a ptisan..and almande mylke, **ordeatum**, i. decoccioun of barly mele. (MED,?a1425 **Chauliac(2)* (MS Paris angl. 25), 95/19)
Tempere hem with **sape**, þat is, swete vynegir y-made of swete wiyn. (Getz, a1475 *GA* (MS Wel 537), 114/20–21)

Semisolid preparations are represented by:

cataplasma (L *cataplasma* 'poultice, plaster'; DMVE and DMLBS, s.v. *cataplasma* n.) 'poultice containing herbs and herbal juices mixed with e.g. flour and grease';
deute (OF/AN *diauté* 'a medicament containing marshmallow'; DMVE, *deute* n., AND, *diauté* n.) 'ointment containing marsmallow roots, linseed and other herbs';
grace (a metaphorical use of OF/AN grace 'gift, power'; DMVE, s.v. *grace* n.) 'some ointment', the name is probably related to another metaphorical name for a medicine *grace of God* 'a plaster used to treat wounds';
gruel (OF/AN *gruel* 'poultice'; DMVE and AND *gruel*) 'poultice, porridge made with medicinal herbs';
magdaleon (OF/AN *magdaliun*, MF *magdaleon*, ML *magdaleo*, CL *magdalia* 'lump of bread used for wiping the hands at the table'; DMVE: s.v. *magdaleon*) 'small cylindrical roll of plaster or some other medicinal substance';
valence/valencia (metaphorical use of L *valentia* 'power, might'; MED s.v. *valence*, DMVE s.v. *valencia*) 'ointment containing herbs and pork fat', cf. also:

(115) **Cataplasma** is, whanne herbis ben grounde & soden ouþer raw (…) & medlid wiþ mele & grese, & it ne schal not be hard ne neische, but in þe meene. (Fleischhacker, a1400 *LSC1* (MS Ashm 1396), 330/28–29)

Deute is þus made: Take of þe rotis of bismalue, þat is, þe hollihock (…) of lynen seed, of femigreke [etc.]. (Getz, a1475 *GA* (MS Wel 537), 102/17–18)

Take old pysse, & boyle hyt, & skem hyt from agalon to aquart, (…) Þys ys þe oynement þat ys cleped **grace**. (Heinrich, c1450 *HRec* (MS Add 33996), 201/24)

Growelles and softe plastres ben as it were þe same, for in **growelles** [**Ch.(1)*: pultez; L pultibus]

(…) þere entreþ but **meles** with water or wiþ Iuses and wiþ oyle or with hony; (MED,?a1425 **Chauliac(2)* (MS Paris angl. 25), 175b/a)

Take þe rotes y-wasshen..be þai riȝt wele cocted in swete water, & be þai stamped, and be þer made **magdalions** [*Ch.(2)*: rolles; L magdaleones]. (MED,?a1425 **Chauliac(1)* (MS NY 12), 170a/a)

Þe fleobotomy y-done, be þer putte vpon of **valence** or some oþer equiualent medicyne. (Power, 1425 *AFS* (MS Sln 6), 70/39)

To the group of semisolid preparations we can also add two preparations used mainly for cosmetic purposes. According to DMVE, *gommery* (ML *gommera*) was a cosmetic ointment or lotion, whereas more commonly recorded *tincture* (L *tinctura*) was a substance for colouring hair or skin. MED adds that *tincture* could have been also used as ointment to cover wounds (DMVE, *gommery* n., MED, *tincture* n.).

There are also a few names for medicaments used to cure eyes, e.g., *burud* (ML < Ar 'eye medicine'), *collyre* (AN/OF *collire*) and *collyrium* (L *collyrium*) 'salve, lotion for eye disorder', and *sief* (ML scief) 'some medical confection for eyes' (DMVE, *burud* n., *collyre* n., *collyrium* n., *sief* n.). The last three names must have been pretty well known as they produced quite a lot of compound forms (e.g. *white collyre, citrine collyrie, resolving collyrie, collyrium album, collyrium rubeum, white sief, sief rosat*, etc.)[77].

The last names to mention are three terms of unknown origin: *colman, sorifilon, verlilium*. The first, *colman*, was recorded in one of texts as an equivalent for *emplastrum nigrum* 'black plaster' (DMVE, a1425 **Chauliac(2)* (MS Jes-C Q.G.23), 389ra: "Emplastrum nigrum.s. colman"). *Sorifilon* 'medicinal preparation against hemoptysis and rectal bleeding' is probably related to L *caryophyllon* 'dried flower-buds of the clove' (cf. DMVE, *sorifilon* n.). The last name, *verlilium*, denoted 'ointment made by boiling litharge, ceruse, calamine, mastic, camphor, rose water, beeswax' (DMVE, *verlilium* n.).

77 For more on these compound forms see the subsections in 5.3; cf. also Appendix B.

5.3 Compounds and phrases

The present section concentrates on 1262 references to medical preparations that have been recorded in the examined sources. The largest group (909 records, 72%) constitute names of Romance origin. These are adoptions of Latin/French names and their translations into Middle English, e.g., *electuarium ducis, emplaster restrictive, oleum de camomille, oil of camomile, pilule de agarico, pilule of agaric*, etc. About 23% (297 records) are hybrid formations, e.g., *emplaster of leeks, syrup of wormwood, water of caprifoil, fleshing medicine, constrictive bath*, etc., and only about 5% (56 records) are represented by combinations including forms of Germanic heritage, e.g., *burning water, dry bath, water of elder, water of honeysuckle*, etc.

The terms under discussion are combinations in which the head noun is a general term for a medicinal preparation (e.g. *medicine*), a term denoting a dosage form (e.g. *ointment, plaster, powder, syrup*), or a term referring to a specific (e.g. *sief, treacle*). Their modifiers specify mostly: (i) the main ingredient of a preparation, (ii) the origin of the medicament, (iii) the affected part of the body or medical condition for which a given mixture is prescribed, and (iv) the properties of a preparation.

As a result, it has been possible to divide the collected examples into the same semantic groups as those established in the section dealing with simplex terms and derivatives. The category "names indicating therapeutic methods" is excluded from this section as the examined material lacks examples that refer to the way a medicament should be administered. The combinations that do not fit in any of the established semantic groups are discussed separately, as miscellaneous names.

5.3.1 Main ingredient(s)

This group includes 600 names for 397 medical preparations. This discrepancy reflects the fact that in Middle English medical writings their compilers, translators or authors, while referring to medical mixtures, often used more than one name. These included adoptions of French and Latin names or their translations into English. As a result, rose oil, one of the most commonly used oils in medical recipes, is recorded with at least ten variant name forms[78]: *oil de roses, oil of rose(s), oil of roset, oil rosarum, oil rosat, oile rose, oil roset, oleum rosaceum, oleum*

78 The list includes the commonest spelling variants. For all spelling variants the available medical writings and dictionaries (DMVE, MED or OED) should be consulted.

rosarum, oleum roses. Likewise, violet oil has six variant names (*oil de violet, oil of violet, oil violet, oleum violace, oleum violaceum, oleum violarum*), alum water has five variant forms (*alum water, alumed water, alumy water, aqua aluminosa, water of alum*), and a plaster containing material from ant-hill and ant eggs has three forms (*emplaster of ants, emplaster of pismires, emplastrum de formicis*), etc. (cf. DMVE, MED, OED and the source texts).

The largest group (541 items, 90%) of names indicating the main ingredients constitute combinations in which the head noun denotes a dosage form, e.g., *oil of mastic, ointment of castor, powder of aloes, syrupus limonum, water of barley*. The remaining 59 examples (10%) are combinations in which the head noun is a name of some specific, e.g., *ciroin of roses, oxymel of radish, sief rosat, treacle diatessaron*. The modifiers of the head nouns form certain semantic groups. Hence, the names under discussion can be divided into three major categories[79]:

(i) combinations in which modifiers specify the ingredient of plant origin, e.g., *ball of fumitory, ciroin of roses, electuary of roses, emplaster of camomile, oil of laurel, ointment of myrtles, oleum nenuphar, pellet of affodil, pilule of euphorbe, powder of aloes, sief rosat, syrup of violet, treacle of asafetida, trochiscus de turbith, unguentum lilium, valence of wormwood, water of plantain*, etc.
(ii) combinations in which modifiers specify the ingredient of animal origin, e.g., *oil of scorpions, ointment of gander, pilule of castor, plaster of worms, potio muscata, powder of castor, unguentum muscatum*, etc.
(iii) combinations in which modifiers specify the ingredient of mineral origin, e.g., *emplaster plumbi, oil of lede, ointment of tutty, oleum tartar, powder of arsenek, sief de plumbo, unguentum de bolo, water of brimstone*, etc.

The first group, the most numerous, contains about 451 names (75% of all instances belonging to the category of names indicating the main ingredients), the second consists of 46 names (8%), and the last of 73 names (12%). There are also 30 (5%) names that could not be included in the above categories. These are, for instance:

(i) 10 names indicating medicaments whose basic ingredient was vinegar[80] combined with other *materia medica* (*emplastrum oxycroceum, oxycratum,*

79 For the full list of names see Appendix B: Compounds and phrases.

80 These are forms with *oxy* derived from ML *oxys* n. 'sharp or vinegar, acid'; in DMLB, *oxys*, adj. and n. Cf. also "**oxi** that is grewe and in latyn Exci is vynegyr" (MEMT, 15th c. *WBMP* (MS Med. Misc. I), 314). For instance, *oxycratum* was a solution of vinegar and water, *oxycroceum* was a plaster containing vinegar and saffron (ML *croceus* 'saffron'),

oxycroceum, oxygranatorum, oxysaccharum, sour syrup, syropus acetosus, syrup of oxymel, syrup of oxysacchare, syrup of vinegar),

(ii) 4 names indicating eggs or egg yolk as the main ingredient (*oil of eggs, oil of ey yolks, oil of eyren* and *water of eyren*),

(iii) 3 names for medicinal water made by leaching ashes (*aqua saponis, water of ashes, water of soap*),

(iv) 2 names denoting a sweet concoction with roses (*rodozacar, rodoraca*)[81], and

(v) 11 examples: *mellicrate* 'medical preparation made by boiling honey mixed with water and/or wine', *oil of man's dirt* 'oil distilled from human feces', *syrupus penidie* 'syrup made with barley sugar', *syrupus julep* 'syrup made by boiling water with sugar' (cf. also DMVE n. *julep* 'sweet medicinal drink prepared by mixing water with sugar' and section 5.2.6), *unguentum de lino/line* and *ointment of line* 'ointment containing lint (ravelled or scraped linen cloth)', *water of cheese* 'whey', *water of man's blood* 'medicinal water made with human blood', *water of a lung* 'medicinal liquid expressed from animal lung', *hiera pigra* 'purgative electuary having aloes as a basic ingredient'.

The last medicament, *hiera pigra*, employed by physicians of ancient Greece and used in medical practice for many centuries later, has a very interesting history[82] as explanations concerning the origin and the meaning are intriguing and vary depending on sources. According to medieval medical texts, *hiera pigra* means 'holy bitter', cf. a Latin version of *Antidotarius Nicholai:* "Yera idest sacra picra idest amara" (DMVE, *hiera pigra* n.) or an explanation in a Middle English translation of the same text "Yera, þat ys to sey, holy. (…) Pigra, þat ys to sey, butre. (…)" (MEMT, 15th c. *AntN* (MS Ferguson 147), f. 53v, f. 37r). This "sacred" name of the medicament probably reflects the fact of the remedy being originally used in some Temples of Asclepius in ancient Greece (cf. Thompson 1929: 36). From OED we can also learn that the name is a combination of Gk *ἱερά* > *hiera* 'sacred', often being an element of the names of Greek pharmaceuticals, and of πίκρα > *pigra* 'bitter (antidote, medicament)' (OED, *hiera picra* n.). According to

---

oxygranatorum was a purgative electuary containing acidic juice from pomegranates (ML *pomum granatum*), and *oxysaccharum* (also MF *oxysacchare*, ML *oxysacchra*) was a syrup made by boiling vinegar and sugar (ML *saccharon, saccarum* 'sugar').

81 Both names are combinations of ML *rhodon* (from Gk ῥόδον) 'rose' and ML *saccharon, saccarum* 'sugar'. Cf. also: "**RODOZACARA**. þat ys to sey, zucarum rosacea, þat ys, sucre roset." (MEMT, 15th c. *AntN* (MS Ferguson 147), f. 40v).

82 For an interesting account on changing formulas for *hiera pigra* throughout history see e.g., Thompson (1929: 35–43).

DMLBS, however, the two words developed other senses: *hiera* 'purgative' and *pigra* 'aloes', hence the MED and DMVE explanations of *hiera pigra* as 'purgative electuary having aloes as basic ingredient'. In Middle English medical writings the medicament is often recorded as either *hiera* or *pigra* (see examples below), both with reference to *hiera pigra*, which suggests that the medicament must have been well known and frequently applied in medical practice, cf.:

(116) Let purge him with **iera** y-medlid with þe poudir of radiche and of yreos. (Getz, a1475 *GA* (MS Wel 537), 148/17)
Þe firste bigynnynge of þis cure is for to avoide þe heed wiþ cochijs & wiþ **pigra**. (Fleischhacker, a1400 *LSC1* (MS Ashm 1396), 253/8)

As regards the structure of the names under discussion, several patterns can be distinguished. The most common pattern (347 examples, 58%) is represented by combinations where the head noun is followed by a genitive *of*-phrase, e.g., *emplaster of mallows, oil of almonde, powder of pigre, water of cauls*, etc. The names are either native formations or translations of Latin terms, cf.:

(117) Þe **emplastre of maluis** [L: emplastrum de malvis (188/11)] is mykel preised. (DMVE, a1425 *Chauliac(1)* (MS Paris angl. 25), 249/29)
Þe **poudre of pigre** [L: pulueris pigre (Z5va)] þat goiþ to þese pelottis.. (Fleischhacker, a1400 *LSC1* (MS Ashm 1396), 183/21)
Medle ham wiþ vynegre and wiþ **water of caules** [L: aqua caulium (84/20)]. (DMVE, a1425 *Chauliac(1)* (MS Paris angl. 25), 110/5)

Apart from the combinations with *of*-phrases there are 55 (9%) records with genitive *de*-phrases, which are mostly anglicised forms of Latin terms, e.g., *emplastrum de arnoglossa, oleum de lilio, unguentum de palma*, etc. A characteristic feature of these names is that the head nouns are usually recorded with the Latin neuter nominative ending *-um* (cf. also 118 below). Other examples constitute adoptions from French and these include, e.g., *oil de ben, oil de bay, oil de laurel, oil de mastic, oil de roses, oil de violet, pellet de agarico*. According to DMVE, one formation, *oil de dill*, is probably a Frenchified version of *oil of dill*, where the name of plant is of Germanic origin recorded in neither French nor Latin (DMVE, *oil* n., *oil de dill*).

(118) Resolue it..wiþ **oleum de been** [L: oleo de ben (357/24)] and with oyle of spyconarde. (DMVE, a1425 *Chauliac(1)* (MS Paris angl. 25), 424/24)
Let it be riped & þe escarre mundified wiþ **emplastrum de apio** [L: emplastro de apio (72/35)]. (DMVE, a1425 **Chauliac(2)* (MS Jes-C Q.G.23), 235ra)

The next pattern (170 examples, 28%) involves combinations where the specifying element (adjective or noun) comes after the head (the so-called Latin/French model)[83], e.g., *emplastrum diaquilon, pilule agaric, pulvis pigre, syrup nenuphar, ointment populeon, oleum anacardinum, unguentum dialthea, water roset,* etc. These names are either adoptions of French/Latin terms or their loan translations, cf.:

(119) He biddeþ ministre þerto medcine mad wiþ..**oile laurin** [L: oleum laurinum (107/13)]. (DMVE, a1425 **Chauliac(2)* (MS Jes-C Q.G.23), 107vb)
The vlcers of þe ȝerde..ben plastrede with þe **oynement populeoun** [L: unguento populeon (464/6)]. (DMVE, a1425 *Chauliac(1)* (MS Paris angl. 25), 637/29)

The least represented (28 examples, 5%) is the Germanic pattern, i.e combinations where the attribute (adjective or noun) is placed before the head noun, e.g., *alumed water, linseed oil, pitchy plaster, plantain water,* etc.

5.3.2 Origin of the preparation

This section concentrates on a group of 148 instances that identify the source of the origin of 99 medical preparations. The largest part of the collected examples (110 records, 78%) constitute combinations with the head noun that denotes a dosage form; in 24 combinations the head noun is a name of some specific, e.g., *diarrhodon abbatis, Galen's ciroin, hierapigra Constantini,* etc., and in 3 records a general term for a medicinal preparation is the head noun, as in *Galen's gladding medicine, Galen's wonderful medicine,* and *medicine of Haly the Abbot.* The remaining 11 examples constitute some figurative expressions for electuaries, ointments or plasters in which the head noun refers to no medicinal form, e.g., *donum Dei* 'gift of God;', *Gratia Dei* 'grace of God', *igia Greca* 'taste of Greece', *virtus a Deo Datum* 'virtue given of God', etc. The modifiers of the head nouns form certain semantic groups, which allows one to divide the material into the following major categories[84]:

(i) combinations in which modifiers specify medical authorities, e.g., *Avicenna's powder, Benvenute's powder, unguentum Rhazes, water of Master Peter, zinziber Alexandrinum,* etc.;
(ii) combinations in which modifiers specify historical figures, e.g., *imperial water, potio Adriani, unguentum agrippa,* etc.;

83 For more on the position of modifiers (especially adjectives) in Middle English nominal phrases and the distinction between so-called Germanic and French-type structures see, for instance, Norri (1989), Raumolin-Brunberg (1994), Moskowich (2002, 2009), Moskowich — Crespo (2002), Fischer (2004, 2006), Sylwanowicz (2016).

84 For the full list of names see Appendix B.

(iii) combinations in which modifiers specify religious or divine (e.g. God) authority, e.g., *emplaster apostolicon, potio Sancti Pauli, theodoricon empericon*, etc.;
(iv) combinations in which modifiers specify place of origin, e.g., *drink of Antioche, French water, Greek powder, plaster of Paris, unguentum Egiptiacum*, etc.

The first group is represented by 71 examples, of which the most numerous are names of preparations attributed to standard Greek and Arab medical authorities (38 records). Galen was an absolute authority for a medieval practitioner, hence his name has been found in at least 11 terms, e.g., *Galen's ciroin, Galen's gladding medicine, Galen's wonderful medicine, Galen's green ointment, Galen's powder, pulvis Galeni, hiera pigra Galeni, leticia Galeni, pilule Gallice*[85], *tiriaca Galeni, unguentum viride Galeni.* Other terms include references to such figures as Andron (a Greek physician to Nero), Atonius Musa (a physician to Roman Emperor Augustus), Alexander of Tralles (a 6th century Byzantine physician), Avicenna (an influential physician and thinker, active in 10th–11th centuries, whose major work, the *Canon*, was used in European and Islamic medical schools till the early modern times), Constantinus Africanus (an 11th century physician and translator of medical writings from Arabic into Latin), Haly (a 10th century physician and psychologist from Persia), Jesus of Haly (= Haram/Ali ibn Isa, an 11th century Arab ophtalmologist), Mesue (an 8th–9th century physician from Persia), Rasis (an outstanding physician and philosopher from Persia, active in 9th–10th centuries), Rufus of Ephesus (a late 1st century Greek physician who wrote on dietetics, pathology and anatomy), and Stephanus (probably Stephanus of Athens, a 6th–7th century philosopher and physician who wrote commentaries on Hippocrates's *Prognostics* and *Aphorisms* and on Galen's *Therapeutics to Glaucon*; Dickson 1998)[86], cf.:

(120) **MUSA ENEA**. Yt haþe his name of þe autor þe wyche compowned. Yt ys [\f. 30r\] god for hem þat haueþ þe feuer tercyan, and þe feuer quarteyne, yȝefe byfore þe hour of acces wyþ hote weyn. (MEMT, 15th c. *AntN* (MS Ferguson 147), f. 29v)

85 According to DMVE *pilule Gallice* is an error form for *pilule Galeni* (cf. DMVE, *pilule Gallice* n.).

86 For more on medical authorities see, for instance, Thompson (1929), Matthews (1962), Getz (1990), Zimmerman — Veith (1993), Jones (1994, 1998b), Porter (2001), Anderson (2005), Wallis (2010), Conrad — Neve et al. (2011), Lindberg — Shank (2015), Zebroski (2016) and www.treccani.it (*Enciclopedia Italiana di Scienze, Lettere ed Arti* i.e. 'Italian Encyclopaedia of Science, Letters, and Arts').

Who so euer forsothe suffren newly vlcers of þe eres..Þo þat be with akþe, cure ham wiþ **pilotes of andronium** [L: trocisci Andromii (237/26)]. (DMVE, a1425 *Chauliac(1)* (MS Paris angl. 25), 317/17)
If þat akþe schulde noye, take þe **oynement of Alisaundre** [L: linimentum Alexandri (464/30)]. (DMVE, a1425 *Chauliac(1)* (MS Paris angl. 25), 638/27)
Couere or hide it wiþ **Avicens powdre** of clowes. (DMVE, a1425 *Chauliac(1)* (MS Paris angl. 25), 478/33)
Medicyns to purgen & to auoyden from þe heuyd ben..**yerapigra Constantini**, yera abbatis. (DMVE, a1414 **Austin* (MS Cai 176/97), 195)
Vnguentum Nigrum haly..is maad of wex, talowʒ and pich & of Galbanum. (DMVE, c1475(1392) *LondonSurg* (MS Wel 564), 290/25)
The **powdre of Haram** [L: pulvis Haram (105/12)], made with þe ryndes of hennes ayren preparate..Iesus appropreþ for to make a seke man slepe. (DMVE, a1425 *Chauliac(1)* (MS Paris angl. 25), 138/8)
Good confecciouns, as is **aromaticon of Hebemesue** [L: aromaticon Hebemesue (351/27) þat is as who seiþ þrosata nouella. (DMVE, a1425 **Chauliac(2)* (MS Jes-C Q.G.23), 316ra)
Þe xij ben mani varie & diuerse & moreouer **puluis Rasis.** Recipe olibanum, aloen, sarcocolle, sancdragoun, þe rote of yreos ana. Let hem be stampid & mad poudre. (DMVE, a1425 **Chauliac(2)* (MS Jes-C Q.G.23), 391va)
If þou anoynte him fro þe nauel dounward, he shal haue deliuerance bineþe. And þe same werking **iera rufa**. (Getz, a1475 *GA* (MS Wel 537), 172/16)
Þis is **vnguentum Stephani** [L: vnguentum Stephanoni (E7vb)] to þe emoroidis. (DMVE, a1475 *PlatearPra* (MS Dd.10.44), 72r)

There is also a medicament attributed to Aristotle – *unguentum Aristotilis* (see 121 below). This can be explained by the fact that this Greek philosopher was seen as an authority in all fields of science, including medicine. In many medieval scholarly works, their authors compare the views of Aristotle and Galen on various medical issues (Siraisi 1990, Pahta — Taavitsainen 1995).

(121) Ane oyntement for all manere of scalles & to gare hare waxe & vocatur **Vnguentum Aristotilis**. (DMVE, c1440 *LiberDivMd* (MS Lin-C 91), 4/4)

Many names are referred to medieval physicians from Italy, such as Benvenutus Grassus (a 13th century author of a popular treatise on eye disorders), Cophon (a 12th century Salernitan physician), Lanfranc of Milan (an influential surgeon; founder of the 14th century French school of surgery), Master Dine (a 13th–14th century physician from Florence, Dino del Garbo), Master Anselm of Genoa (a 13th century surgeon), Matthaeus Platearius (a 12th century scholar from Salerno), Master William Someries (prob. Guliamo Corvi – a friend of Lanfranc, cf. Fleischhacker 1894: 348) or Theodoric (a 13th century surgeon from the Bologna School), cf.:

(122) Þe 5e is put **Beneuentis poudre** [L: pulvis Benevenuti (461/22)] ..for al spottis. (DMVE, a1425 **Chauliac(2)* (MS Jes-C Q.G.23), 406ra)

ȝif þe cause be hote as in hote feueris, recipe electuari patris mei, **electuari Cophonis** [etc.]. (DMVE, a1414 **Austin* (MS Cai 176/97), 219)

Þe lesse wondeȝ..cured I with vnguento viridi, i.*[e.] **grene oyntment of lanfrank**. (Power, 1425 *AFS* (MS Sln 6), 54/3)

Þe firste is **Maistre Dynes powdre** [L: pulvis magistri Dini (462/15–16)], þat is: Take of scrophularie..of gynger.. of brian, of pilettre, of wodebynde [etc.]. (DMVE, a1425 *Chauliac(1)* (MS Paris angl. 25), 635/22)

The fifte fourme is the **chief plastre of Maister Anselme of Ianuaye** [L: emplastrum capitale magistri Anserini de Ianua (459/41–42)] and draweþ oute quittre. (DMVE, a1425 *Chauliac(1)* (MS Paris angl. 25), 632/5)

I made hem **a sirupe of platearie** in þis maner/ ℞, succiscariole (…). (Fleischhacker, a1400 *LSC1* (MS Ashm 1396), 286/6)

Also an **oynement þat Maister William Someris made**/ ℞, rasinam albam & liquefactam (…). (Fleischhacker, a1400 *LSC1* (MS Ashm 1396), 348/15–16)

Let leye þer vpon a plagelle **Thederikis liniment** made of ious of lunarie & planteyn wiþ sal gemme. (DMVE, a1425 **Chauliac(2)* (MS Jes-C Q.G.23), 217 va)

There are also medicaments named after French medical masters, such as Master Petrus de Bonato (a 14th century surgeon at Lyons, probably a friend of Guy de Chauliac, cf. DMVE), Master Arnald de Villanova (a 13th/14th century physician; translated a number of medical books from Arabic) and Walter of Agilon (a 13th century master of medicine at Montpellier, cf. O'Boyle 1998: 113), cf.:

(123) The fourþe fourme is þe grene **plastre of Maistre Pers de Bonaunt** [L: emplastrum viride magistri Petri de Bonant (438/22–23)]. (DMVE, a1425 *Chauliac(1)* (MS Paris angl. 25), 601/11)

In þe fourþe, is putte **Maistre Arnaldes powdre**, drieng teres and amendynge þe redenesse..Take tutie..of antymoyne..of margery perles [etc.]. (DMVE, a1425 *Chauliac(1)* (MS Paris angl. 25), 634/10)

Take iiij penyweyȝte of scamony..and iij penywheyȝte of **poudre Wauter**. (DMVE, c1475 **ThesPauper* (MS Sln 1764), 25r)

One preparation is attributed to 13th century Master Peter of Spain (Petrus Hispanicus, later Pope John XXI), who is known for a treatise on eye diseases, while another medicament carries the name of an English surgeon, John of Bradmore, who was active in the late 14th and 15th century; Lang (1998), Daly - Yee (2001), cf.:

(124) To þe same entencioun beþ the water of fenel, of rewe..and þe preciouse **water of Maystre Petre** [L: aqua preciosa magistri Petri Hyspani (346/14)]. (DMVE, a1425 *Chauliac(1)* (MS Paris angl. 25), 470/26)

Leye þerto **Emplastrum ffuscum Brademore**. (DMVE, c1475(1392) *LondonSurg* (MS Wel 564), 288/1)

Sometimes, reference is not made to a name of a particular author but to a group of medical experts (see examples under 125) or to a medical writing, such as *Liber ad Almasoris* by Rhazes, cf. *unguentum viride Almasoris* (DMVE, *unguentum* n.).

(125) Hele vp þi wounde with **vnguentum viride cirurgicorum**. (DMVE, a1450 **Mond&ChSurg* (MS Sln 2463), 71v)
The **oynement of þe Foure Maysters** [L: unguentum quatuor magistrrum (233/39)] is special in þat þat it is made of mynte, of egrimoyne, of oculus christi and of verueyne ybeten wiþ swynes grece. (DMVE, a1425 *Chauliac(1)* (MS Paris angl. 25), 312/15)

Apart from medical authorities, there are 12 names which reflect the names of historical characters. These are references to ancient kings or emperors, such as Agrippa, Hadrian or Justinian the Great (cf. also the discussion of *adrianum*, *agrippa* and *iustinum* in section 5.2.2), cf.:

(126) In þis oinement in anoþer place it semeþ þat Thederik addeþ þe herbes þat gon into vnguentum arogon & **vnguentum agrippa**. (DMVE, a1425 **Chauliac(2)* (MS Jes-C Q.G.23), 149va)
ȝif þis accesse comeþ in heuest, he shalle be made hole wiþ drenkes þat bien yclepid **pocio Adriani** & diacalamenti. (DMVE, a1475 **ExperDinam* (MS Bl Add. 34111), 158r)
For þe stone in þe blader..An drenk þat is clepid **pocio Iustini** idronk wiþ hote wyne helpeþ mochel. (DMVE, a1475 **ExperDinam* (MS Bl Add. 34111), 142r)
ELECTUARIUM DUCIS. Yt ys of an abbot on court þe wyche compowned this lectuarye for nede of duk Robert. Ys ys good for indigestioun and ventosyte of þe stomake and of þe entrels, and to ache of þe boctokes, and for yuele of þe stone. (MEMT, 15th c. *AntN* (MS Ferguson 147), f. 19v)

The last medicament in the quotations above, although attributed to Roger, Duke of Apulia, is said to have been prepared by Abbas Curiae, a chaplain of the royal household; cf. also DMVE, *electuarium ducis* n. Another cure ascribed to Abbas is *diarrhodon abbatis* 'an electuary containing roses and syrup of roses' (DMVE, *diarrhodon* n.).

In one medical text the translator renders L *oleum regium* 'king's oil' as *Kynge Wylleham oyle* 'King William oil' (DMVE, a1475 *PlatearPra* (MS Dd.10.44), 96va). Considering the fact that the translation was made in the second half of the 15th century (i.e. the time of King Edward's IV rule), it is difficult to state with certainty to whom a given medicament was actually attributed.

In some combinations, such as *diarrhodon Julii* 'electuary containing roses and attributed to some Julius' (DMVE, *diarrhodon* n.), it is difficult to identify the author of the medicament. There are also examples with general references that imply that a medicament is attributed to or used by the members of the royalty, cf.:

(127) The seuenþe is þe **Kynges oynement** [L: unguentum regis Anglie (438/39–40)]: Take of white wexe, of rosyn..of oyle..of waschen terebentyne..of frank ensence, of mastik..make þerof an oynement. (DMVE, a1425 *Chauliac(1)* (MS Paris angl. 25), 601/34)
A preciose water emonge all waters (…) it [is] clepid **water emperiall** ffor all emperoures and grote lordis emonge the sarsyns vse to drynke it. (DMVE, c1450 *RemLMSoc.* (MS Wel 136), 298/32)
Whan þat cold materie ys digeste, þanne purge it with..**katarticum ymperiale**. (DMVE, a1414 **Austin* (MS Cai 176/97), 215)

The first is defined as 'ointment containing beeswax, rosin, olive oil, turpentine, frankincense, mastic' (DMVE, *King's oinement* n.), the second is 'medicinal water distilled from four plants: tormentil, dittany of Crete or white dittany, field scabious or small scabious (…), scarlet pimpernel' (DMVE, *imperial water* n.), whereas the last preparation is an 'electuary purging several humours (choler, melancholy, salty phlegm)' (DMVE, *catharticum imperiale* n.)

The third group of names to be considered are combinations with references to religious or divine (i.e. God or gods) entities. Altogether 28 examples have been recorded. These include combinations with *apostolicon*, *Esdra* and *theodoricon*, the names that have already been discussed in section 5.2.2 concerning simplex terms and derivations.

To the names that attribute the medicament to God belong *donum Dei*, *emplastrum Gratia Dei* (also recorded as *grace of God*, *Gratia Dei*, *Gratia Dei maior*, *Gratia Dei media*, *more gratia Dei*), *virtue given of God*, *virtus a Deo datum*. In the recipe for a plaster called *donum Dei* 'gift of God' there is a comment on the origin of the name, being at the same time an explanation about the importance of God in medical practice, cf.:

(128) A playstir whiche is callyd **donum dei**..hath his name of effecte and his goodnesse, <u>for it is bettir mad of God þanne of man</u>, and it helyth all woundys. (DMVE,?c1450 *StockhRec* (MS Stockh 10.90), 129/4)

Another plaster, *Gratia Dei* 'grace of God', has its name from a legend which says that "an angel brought it down from heaven to King Alexander for the people of his land, when they were all near lost with deadly woundes of spear, dart, and dagger, and with many other maladyes as the surgeons have long since fayned."

(Thompson 1929: 165). *Gratia Dei* was also a name of a herb[87] which, surprisingly, was not used in the preparation of the plaster carrying the same name. Compare the following fragments with a description of a herb and a recipe for the plaster:

(129) **Gratia dei** is an herbe þat men clepe, gratia dei. Þis herbe haȝt lewys lyk to þe dendelyoun. but þelewys of þis herbe arn sumdel scharpe and it haȝt a ȝelwȝ flour and it growyth in drye ground. (MEMT, a1450 *ACH* (MS Roy-L 10.90), 161)
Medcyn þat is called **Gratia Dei**, þat is made on þis manere: Tak litarge iiij vnces, ceruse iij vnces, roste of a belle of bras ij vnces, of vertgres ij vnces, of sarcocol iiij vnces, of mastik, galbanum, ammoniak, of ilkane iiij vnces, with encence iij vnces, of bedellium halfe ane vnce, of pik greke, pik nauill, of þam ij vnces. (…) **This emplaster** clenses wondis and sowdis þam to-gedir & dose owte dede flesche & newe flesche gars grewe. It is a gud heler for brynnand werkes, wondis & kiles, whare so bee. (MEMT, 1440 *LDM* (MS Thornton A.5.2), 68)

There is also an ointment, *virtue given of God* or *virtus a Deo datum*, whose quality and advantage over other medicaments was due to its being a gift from God, cf.:

(130) Þanne þe medicine schal be putte withinne þe ye þe weche is callyd **virtus a Deo datum**, þat is to seye a **vertyw yoven of God** [L: virtus a Deo datum (35v)].. For þe grete vertyw it hath in werkynge it is callyd so tofore alle oþer medicines. (DMVE, a1425 *Arderne(3)* (MS Em 69), 69v)

Some terms attribute medical preparations to Biblical figures (angels, Mary Magdalene, Nicodemus who brought embalming ointment for Jesus's body, Saint Paul), mythological figures (Hermes and Venus), and one is ascribed to some Bishop of Laudun (France), cf.:

(131) Tak þe leues of spourge and.. ȝucre, gynger & flour of whete mele, & mak paste & bake it..& þu sal haue deliuerance bathe abown & bynethe. Þis is called **angell brede**. (DMVE, c1440 *LiberDivMd* (MS Lin-C 91), 28/1)
Here is þe **oynement of Marie Magdaleine**. Take saueye & cipris & rose marie, (…). (DMVE, c1450 **RemSl.* (MS Sln 3153), 54v)
<**Vnguentum Nichodemi**> Recipe mirre, aloes, sarcocolle (…). (DMVE, c1475(1392) *LondonSurg* (MS Wel 564), 386/2)
Diacastoreum and **pocio Sancti Pauli** with wyn of rewe..cureþ epilence. (DMVE, c1450 *Theodoric(1)* (MS Pep 1661), 170)
Special medicynes to torturam biþ þese: **yera heremetes** [L: yera hermetis (h3vb)]. (DMVE, c1425 **BernLiliyum* (MS Ashm 1505), 93v)

87 *Gratia Dei* (also L *Gratiola*) was a name of hedgehyssop (cf. Gerard's *Herbal*, first published in 1597 and revised in 1633 by Thomas Johnson (Gerard 2015 [1633]: 582).

Vnguentum veneris, ouþer vnguentum apostolorum..is good for to remeue awei fleisch in vlceris. (Fleischhacker, a1400 *LSC1* (MS Ashm 1396), 342/1)
Þe **Bisshoppes oynement** of Laudune [L: unguentum episcopi Laudunensis (442/11)]..Take of swynes grece..of quyk siluer quenchede with spatil (…). (DMVE, a1425 *Chauliac(1)* (MS Paris angl. 25), 606/34)

The next group of names (32 records) comprises combinations which indicate a place of origin of a medicament. Most names include references to the places that are associated with Greek and Arab world of medicine (cf. 132a). The remaining examples (132b) denote European countries or towns, many of them being centres of medical learning, such as Montpellier or Salerno[88], cf.:

(132) a. Also **pillule arabice** ycompouned aȝen þe hed ache ȝif hym vij or ix. (DMVE, c1450 *Theodoric(1)* (MS Pep 1661), 75)
Puluis grecus [L: puluis Grecus (56v)] is þus made: Recipe auripigment, citrin, piper, nigi, calcis viue (…). (Power, 1425 *AFS* (MS Sln 6), 92/8)
b. Þe **plastre of Mounpilers** is a special þing þerin of reed colis soden wiþ lie of wood aschis (…). (DMVE, a1425 **Chauliac(2)* (MS Jes-C Q.G.23), 407ra)
(…) and when he goyth to bede lete hym resceyue of our electuarye clepyd **dyaolibanum Salernitanum** tyl he be hole. (MEMT, 1474–1499 *BG* (MS Hunter V.8.6), 68)

There are some names that fit none of the already discussed semantic categories. For instance, *fellow's water* 'medicinal water for eye troubles' was a form used in John of Gaddesden's *Rosa Anglica*[89] (DMVE, *water* n., *fellow's water*). However, it is not known whether the element *fellow* refers here to a friend of Gaddesden to whom the medicament is attributed. It is possible that by using the form *fellow* 'close, good companion; a chap' (MED, *felaue* n.) the author of the term wanted to evoke positive connotations for the prescribed medicament. Another medicament, an electuary 'against consumptive overheating and loss of moisture' was referred to as: *electuarium patris*, *electuarium patris mei* or *my father's electuary*, all being translations of L *electuarium patris (nostri)* (DMVE, *electuarium* n. and *electuary* n.). This time there is no explanation concerning who might have been the author of the medicament. But it may have been a fairly well-known medicament as the references were documented in two different sources, cf.:

88 For more on European centres of medical learning see, for instance, Matthews (1962), Siraisi (1990), Garcia-Ballester et al. (1994), Porter (2001), Zebroski (2016).

89 John Gaddesden was an English physician active in 13th–14th centuries. He was "so far as is known, the first Englishman who was Court physician to an English monarch" and the author of a treatise on medicine known as *Rosa Anglica*, though the author himself titled it *Rosa Medicinae* (Cholmeley 1912: 3).

(133) Hereto helpiþ nameliche an eleccuarie þat hatte **electuarium patris** [L: electuarium patris (13va)]. (DMVE, a1425(1398) *BarthPopr* (MS Bl Add. 27944), 383/26)
ȝeue þe pacient yt **my fadere electuare** [L: electuraium patris mei (E2rb)] to þe restoringe of þe moysthede. (DMVE, a1475 *PlatearPra* (MS Dd.10.44), 37r)

The names discussed in this section, similarly to the material presented in 5.3.1, exhibit four major structural patterns. Combinations with the head noun followed by a genitive *of*-phrase are fairly well represented (40 examples, 27%). In the texts, these combinations are either translations of the forms used in French/Latin source texts or explanatory terms of foreign forms used in the Middle English medical compilations, cf.:

(134) The fifte fourme is the chief **plastre of Maister Anselme of Ianuaye** [L: emplastrum capitale magistri Anserini de Ianua (459/41–42)] and draweþ oute quittre. (DMVE, a1425 *Chauliac(1)* (MS Paris angl. 25), 632/5)
Þe lesse wondeȝ..cured I with vnguento viridi, i. *[e.] **grene oyntment of lanfrank** [L: vnguento viridi de Launfranc (95r)]. (Power, 1425 *AFS* (MS Sln 6), 54/3)

In contrast to the names indicating the main ingredient(s), the present material contains no combinations with the head followed by the Latin/French *de*-phrases. Instead, there are a number of forms with English *s*-genitive (23 examples, 15%), cf.:

(135) Þe fourtþe forme is **Galiens grene oynement** [L: unguentum viride Galieni (440/7–8)]..Take oyle, of wexe..melte ham..putte þerto of vertegrece. (DMVE, a1425 *Chauliac(1)* (MS Paris angl. 25), 603/31)
Rasis white plastre is gode for alle hote sores & olde sores. Take ofe ceruse.. ofe white wax [etc.]. (DMVE, c1425 **RemSl.* (MS Sln 73b), 184v)

Although the periphrastic genitive was the most frequent variant used in Middle English noun phrases[90], the use of *s*-genitive in the combinations indicating the authors of medicaments is of no surprise, as this variant was usually used with modifiers that designated personal nouns (cf. Wełna 1996: 83).

90 According to Fries (1938, 1940) by 1300 the *of*-construction was the most frequent variant form and increased to about 85% (cf. also a summary of his findings in Yngve 1975). For more on the development of the periphrastic phrase in later centuries see also Biber — Clark (2002) and their analysis of the development of a postmodification pattern in the medical writings across centuries (17th–20th) which shows that *of*-phrases were more frequent than phrases with other prepositions. Similar findings are presented in Raumolin-Brunberg's (1991) examination of the post-modifying prepositional phrases in the 16th century prose of Sir Thomas More.

As regards combinations in which the head is preceded by a modifier other than *s*-genitive, only 8 instances have been recorded. In these combinations, the pre-modifier specifies mostly the colour of the medicament denoted by a head noun, and the information concerning the origin/authorship of the preparation is expressed by an *of*-phrase, cf.:

(136) To þe same entencion vailiþ þe **blac poudre of Arnald** þat schal be seid in þe antidotarie. (DMVE, a1425 **Chauliac(2)* (MS Jes-C Q.G.23), 296ra)

The largest part (84 examples, 57%) constitute combinations that are adoptions of the so-called Latin/French model, cf.:

(137) **Vnguentum Egipciacum**..is made wiþ verdegrece, wiþ alume and wiþ hony and wiþ vynegre. (DMVE, a1425 *Chauliac(1)* (MS Paris angl. 25), 99/4).
Medicyns componyd for þe same doyngge ben þese: **katarticum ymperiale**, diasene..**theodoricon ymperiston**. (DMVE, a1414 **Austin* (MS Cai 176/97), 191)

5.3.3 Parts of the body or health condition

This group comprises combinations in which the modifiers indicate either an affected part of the body or an ailment for which a given medicament is prescribed. Although the names could be divided into two separate semantic groups (names indicating part of the body and names indicating a health condition), they are discussed in the same section as there are only 18 instances (two of which identify also the inventor of the medicament, i.e.: *emplaster capital of Master Anselm of Genoa* and *chief plaster of Anselm of Genoa*, discussed in the previous section). In 15 formations the head nouns denote dosage forms, whereas in 3 cases the head noun is expressed by a general term *medicine.*

The largest part constitute names indicating part of the body (14 examples) to be cured. They are names of medicaments for:

(i) head injuries: *capital medicine, capital plaster, plaster capital, capital powder, pulvis capitalis, chief powder,* and two examples attributed to Master Anselm of Genoa,
(ii) nerves and tendons: *emplaster nerval, emplastrum nerval, unguentum nerval* (cf. also the discussion of *nerval* in section 5.2.3),
(iii) stomach problems: *powder of stomaticon comfortativum, pulvis stomaticus comfortativus,*
(iv) a particular part of the body (usually specified in the text): *medicyns þat ben particuler.*

The remaining five examples concern medicaments for non-chronic sickness (*acute medicine*), a pill against arthritis or gout (*pilule artetice*), two potions for wounds (*potio vulneratorum* < L *vulnero* 'to wound', DMLBS) and *wounded men's drink*, and a plaster for cleaning wounds (*emplaster sanguiboetos*)[91].

As regards the structural patterns of the combinations under discussion, most names are either adoptions of the Latin/French (8 examples) or Germanic patterns (5 examples). There are 3 instances with the *of*-phrase (*chief plaster of Anselm of Genoa, emplaster capital of Master Anselm of Genoa, powder of stomaticon comfortativum*), one record with *s*-genitive (*wounded men's drink*), and one formation in which the head noun is followed by a *that*-clause (*medicyns þat ben particuler*).

5.3.4 Properties of the preparation

This group is represented by 475 names of about 410 preparations that have been recorded in the material examined for the present study. As in previous sections, the collected examples are mostly combinations in which the head noun is a general term for a medicament (170 records, about 36%), e.g., *medicine generative, medicine apertive, rotting medicine*, etc., a term indicating a dosage form (265 records, about 55%), e.g., *breaking ointment, burning water, emplaster resolutive, syrup digestive*, etc., and a name of some specific (38 records, 8%), e.g., *citrine sief, cold diapapaver, oxymel laxativum, stomaticon frigidum*, etc. The remaining two examples include metaphorical references to some ointments: *vade mecum* (L 'go with me', 'all-purpose remedy'; DMVE, *vade mecum* n., DMLBS, *vademecum* n.) and *veni mecum* (L 'come with me'; DMVE, *veni mecum* n.). The modifiers indicate a characteristic feature of a medicament expressed by the head noun.

The largest group (347 examples, 73%) is represented by combinations in which modifiers indicate "drugs' actions" i.e. 'ways of remedying various conditions; healing properties'. The examples collected for this section are classified into the same semantic groups as the simplex terms discussed in section 5.2.5. Below follows a list of selected examples[92]:

(i) closing medicines: *binding medicine, fleshing ointment, unguentum consolidativum*, etc.;

(ii) constricting medicines: *strictory medicine, restraining powder, syrupus stypticus*, etc.;

(iii) opening medicines: *medicine aperitive, oil diaphoretic, unstopping powder*, etc.;

91 For more on this plaster see the discussion in 5.2.3.

92 The full list of terms is presented in Appendix B.

(iv) cleansing medicines: *abstersive medicine, plaster mundificative, cleansing powder*, etc.;
(v) purging medicines: *medicine attractive, drawing medicine, oinement laxative*, etc.;
(vi) repercussive medicines: *emplaster repercussive, medicine consumptive, plaster wasting*, etc.;
(vii) corrosive medicines: *ardent water, medicine cauterative, ointment ruptory*, etc.;
(viii) dissolving medicines: *emplaster dissolutive, loosing medicine, plaster resolutive*, etc.;
(ix) reducing medicines: *subtiliative medicine, subtling medicine*;
(x) drying medicines: *emplaster dessicative, drying oinement, medicine siccative*, etc.;
(xi) moistening medicines: *electuary humiditative, medicine humectative, moist ointment*, etc.;
(xii) suppurative medicines: *maturative medicine, riping emplaster*, etc.;
(xiii) palliative medicines: *abating medicine, comfortable drink, oil mitigative*, etc.;
(xiv) mollifying medicines: *neshing medicine, oinement mollificative, soft plaster*, etc.;
(xv) heating medicines: *chafing medicine, medicine heating*, etc.;
(xvi) cooling medicines: *electuary frigidum, keeling medicine, stomaticon frigidum*, etc.;
(xvii) preventive medicines: *medicine defensive, powder conservative*, etc.;
(xviii) restorative medicines: *emplaster restorative, ointment sanative*, etc.;
(xix) alterative medicines: *changing medicine, drink alterative, syrup alterative*, etc.

Apart from the names that describe healing properties, there are examples that point at other distinctive attributes of medical preparations. For instance, names indicating the quality of the medicament (*cold medicine, dry syrup, hot electuary, temporate medicine*, etc.). These names allude to the theory of the four humours which provided framework for explaining diseases and their causes. The drugs were to counterbalance the excess of one of the humours (blood, phlegm, yellow bile and black bile). For instance, yellow bile had, according to that theory, hot and dry qualities. Thus, its excess would be treated with cold and moist remedies[93].

93 For more on humoral theory see, for instance, Cartwright (1986: 3–4), Porter (2001: 68, 92), Ackerknecht (2016). See also a discussion in sections 2.2 and 5.2.5 of this study.

The next group comprises general labels for preparations that today might be referred to as topical medications, i.e. those applied to a particular place in or on the body, e.g., *local medicine, medicine to the place, adjutorium locale, adjutorium to the place, adjutory to the place* (DMVE n. *adjutorium* from L *adiutorium* 'help, remedy').

There are also two names (*chirurgical medicine, physical medicine*) which show that there was a distinction between medicaments used in surgery and those used in general medical practice, cf.:

(138) Eueryche **medicyn**, or it ys **fisical or cirurgical** or diete. (DMVE, a1414 **Austin* (MS Cai 176/97), 148)
Capitulum 8m of sundi grees of **cirurgical medicyns**. (DMVE, a1425 **Chauliac(2)* (MS Jes-C Q.G.23), 20ra)

Some names specify a colour of the medicament (*black emplaster, citrine ointment, green ointment, unguentum nigrum*, etc.), or its flavour/aroma (*aqua aromatica, electuarium dulce*, etc.).

Several terms are labels for waters obtained through the infusion of herbs (*infused water*) or distillation (*distilled water, stilled water, first water, second water* and *third water*). The numbers, first, second, third, indicate the kind of liquid that condenses during distillation. According to the sources these waters differed also in colour. Thus, "Þe ferste water wol be like to gold, þe secounde as seluer, þe þridde as baume." (Heinrich, c1450 *HRec* (MS Add 33996), 102/5). The most popular and commonly used liquid medication obtained through distillation was known as *aqua vite* or *water of life*. These two terms, however, are a bit misleading as they were labels for alcoholic distillates, usually obtained from distilled wine to which herbs and spices were often added, cf.:

(139) For to makyn **aqua vite**, Fylle a potte of old reed wyn, and doo þere-inne powdir of canell, gyllofre, gingefere, peletre, notemuge, ganyngale [23 spices and herbs listed] ..Stylle it with soft fyir. (DMVE,?c1450 *StockhRec* (MS Stockh 10.90), 27/1)

From some sources we can also learn that the real *aqua vite* is the one that drops first during the distillation process, cf.:

(140) Forto make **aqua vite** that is parfit and worchith many merueiles..Take of terbentyne [etc.]. Distille hem first with an esy fire and afterwarde with grettere. An the first that rennyth is aqua vite. (DMVE, **RemTrin.* (MS Trin-C O.8.35), 111r and 111v)

There are also names which place emphasis on the fact that some medicaments are outstanding. These include combinations in which the head noun is modified by evaluating adjectives, e.g., *precious ointment* and *unguentum preciosum*, *oinement of gleyr* and *unguentum glorie, unguentum speciale, oil bennet* and *oleum benedictum, benedicta potio, pulvis benedictus/benedicte*[94], *great treacle, treacle maior, tricata magna, tiriaca maior, pulvis pliris* (ML *pliris* 'complete, principal', cf. AntN 67 "Pliris est completa medicina", DMVE n. *pliris*), *powder sine pari, pulvis sine pari*[95] (L *sine pari* 'without equal; peerless').

In addition, there are names of the preparations that could be labelled as 'all-purpose medicines'. For instance, *universal medicine* was a name of a medication or cure for sicknesses in a variety of body parts (cf. DMVE, *univeral medicine*). Another term, *vade mecum* 'go with me', which is today associated with manuals or guidebooks, in medieval medical writings was recorded with the sense 'all-purpose remedy' and was used with reference to an ointment (*unguentum vade mecum*). Similarly, *veni mecum* 'come with me' was a label for an ointment containing similar ingredients as *unguentum vade mecum* (DMVE, *vade mecum* n. and *veni mecum* n.).

If we consider the structure of the combinations examined in this section, two patterns are prevalent: (i) formations with the head noun preceded by an adjective (257 records, 54%), a Germanic pattern, and (ii) formations with the head noun followed by an adjective (187, 39%), a Latin/French pattern. The remaining names include some instances with the *of*-phrase (e.g. *oil of styptic, ball of calidicon, ointment of gleyr, pellet of calidicon, powder of calidicon, powder of stomaticon comfortativum*) and with the head noun followed by the infinitive or *that*-phrase (e.g. *adjutorium to the place, adjutory to the place, emplaster þat is mitigative, oinement þat is keeling, medicine þat beþ consuming, medicine to the place*, etc.).

5.3.5 Miscellaneous names

This section contains names (altogether 23) that neither fit in with the four major categories discussed earlier nor betray their meaning as plainly as other examples. Although some of these terms might have been obvious for an experienced physician, they were not necessarily clear to anyone outside the profession. Thus, one must often read thoroughly the text of a recipe in order to find out what sort of medicament these terms refer to.

---

94 See also the discussion of *benedicta* in section 5.2.4.

95 According to the sources this powder was created by Arderne, cf.: "(…) my poudre þat I, Iohn Arderne, made, whiche I called 'puluer sine pari,' an[d] on frenssh, 'poudre saunȝ pere.' I wist neuer, forsoþe, ne knew poudre like to it, (…)." (Power, 1425 *AFS* (MS Sln 6), 26/20–23).

The first group of examples to consider are names which specify the number of ingredients. Some of these reflect a common medieval division of medicaments into simple (made of one basic ingredient) and compound (more than one ingredient)[96], e.g., *aqua composita, simple medicine, compound medicine, compound electuarium, electuarium pluris, oxymel compositum, oxymel compound, oxymel simplex, simple oil.* To this group we can add formations in which the modifier of the head noun provides information on the exact number of ingredients a medicament is composed of, e.g., *unguentum tetrapharmacum* 'ointment made of four ingredients', *pilule optomere* or *pilule octomere* 'pills made of eight ingredients' (DMVE).

Another group of preparations includes such examples as *aqua salutis* (L *salus* 'health'; DMVE, *aqua salutis* n.) 'medicinal water made by boiling tanning liquor, alum, and madder', *balneum eucratum* 'medicated bath restoring the balance between humours' (ML *eucrasia* 'good composition, good temperament'; DMVE, *balneum eucratum* n.), *lac virgineum* (L 'maiden's milk'; DMVE, *lac virgineum* n.) 'milk-like liquid prepared by dissolving litharge in vinegar and adding salt solution', *water of iron* (also *ironed water* and *smith's water*) 'water in which blacksmith has plunged heated iron for cooling' (cf. DMVE, *water* n.).

Some names, such as *powder creoferoberon* (also *powder of creoferoberon, pulver creoferoberon*) and *salus populi* have been recorded only in the writings of Arderne, which suggests that they might have not been well known and hence required some explanation. The first three forms denote a powder used to remove excessive formation of granulation tissue which was made from verdigris, vitriol, orpiment, alum (see 141a; DMVE, *powder* n.). The next medication, *salus populi* (L *salus populi*, literally 'safety of people'; DMLBS, *salus* n. and *populus* n.) was, as the quotation below suggests (141b), some drying ointment, cf.:

(141) a. <The **pouder of creoferoberon** [L: puluis creoferoboron (84v)]> In þe myddell of þe wounde þer appered grete bygges of flessch..A poudir for þe seyde tetys or bygges þat is callyd creoferoberon. Take vertegrece, vitriole, orpiment, alum ana. (DMVE, a1425 *Arderne(3)* (MS Em 69), 169v)

b. **Salus populi**..dryeþ wele and sicatrizeþ, and it availeþ at þe best to lippez ybrent of þe sone or chynned of þe wynde. (Power, 1425 *AFS* (MS Sln 6), 91/6)

There is also a special use of the term *sanc dragans*. According to MED (*sandragoun* n.) and OED (*sandragon* n.), the term, originally OF *sanc de dragon*, ML *sanguis dragonis*, denoted 'the red juice or resin of the dragon tree' or 'a sweetened pottage named for the color produced by adding this red juice'. In DMVE

96 This division is discussed in more detail earlier in chapter two.

(*sanc dragans* n.), however, we can find a quotation which records the term as a label for some ointment, cf.:

(142) Take an cranes heed and þe feete & bray hem in a mortar. And take talough and virgyne wax and temper alle togeder. And **þis salue ys clepyd sank dragans**. (DMVE, c1450 **RemTrin.* (MS Trin-C R.14.51), 5v)

5.4 Distribution of terms denoting specifics in three types of texts: remedy books, surgical texts and specialised treatises

The data in the previous sections demonstrate that Middle English could boast of numerous references to medical specifics. However, numerous as they were, the terms varied in their use and distribution in texts representing different writing traditions. The present section offers a discussion of findings concerning the general tendencies of the use of the names of specifics in the three types of medical writings, i.e. remedy books, surgical works and specialised treatises. Special attention will be paid to items common to all texts and those peculiar to one type of a text. Next, it will be seen how the compilers/writers differed in the use of forms of different etymology, and how they managed to facilitate the understanding of not-yet-familiar foreign terms.

The material used in the following analysis consists of examples extracted from the medical writings examined for the present study[97]. Altogether, 1119 references to about 1032 medical preparations have been identified in these texts. The relative normalized frequency of references to medicaments in different types of medical writings is shown in Figure 7.

97 The material is described in chapter one, section 1.5 (texts included in MEMT and text editions).

Fig. 7: The relative normalized frequency (RNF per 100,000 words) of the names of specifics in the analysed material

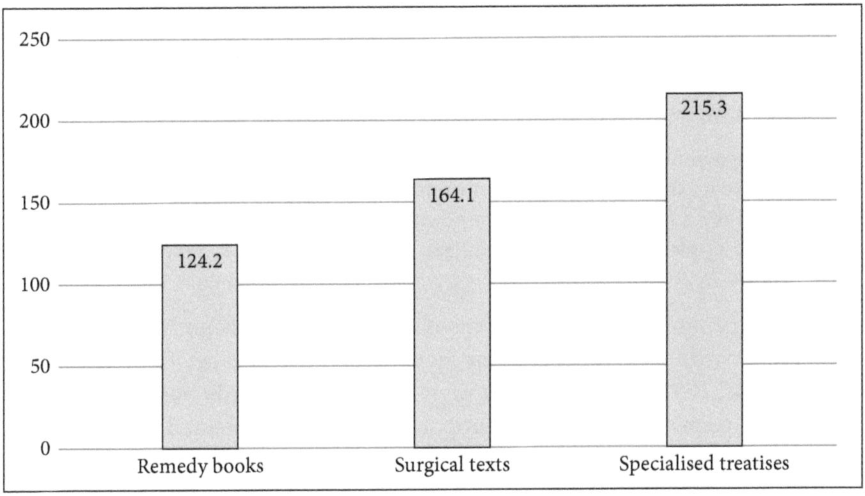

The terms under study are prevalent in texts representing a more learned register (i.e. surgical and specialised texts, RNF: 164.1 and 215.3 respectively). In remedy books, on the other hand, the amount of the terms seems remarkably small (RNF: 124.2), especially if we consider the fact that these texts consist mostly of the collections of recipes. In the material examined for the present study, out of about 2823 recipes extracted from the three collections of texts 82% have been recorded in remedy books, and only 10% in surgical writings and 8% in specialised treatises. Thus, one would expect more references to the names of medicaments in the remedybook collections. The data, however, suggest that the use of the terms, especially references to medical specifics, largely depended on the level of the text (learned and non-learned) but not on its content.

A relatively infrequent use of labels for medicaments in remedy books might be accounted for by the fact that these texts were often accessed by lay readers. These collections were regarded as handbooks for consultation, i.e. their main role was to serve as quick reference books (Taavitsainen 2001). It was necessary to make sure that the potential user of the medical manual would easily find a cure for various ailments. For instance, starting a recipe with *For alcalcolon* or just a name of the medicament *Alcalcolon* 'a compound medicine against tertian fever' might have been meaningless and not very informative for an inexperienced reader. Hence, the use of statements of purpose: *For/Against tertian fever* or *Medicine against fever*, seemed a better solution. Therefore, in these texts, especially in the headings of the recipes[98], instead of the names of pharmaceuticals, there prevail references to a medical problem. In the examined material 87% of the headings of all recipe instructions recorded in remedy books consist of statements of purpose. In the remaining cases, when the name of the medicament occurs it is often translated (especially if a term is of Latin origin) and supplemented with an explanation which ailments could be treated with the use of the preparation it refers to, cf.:

(143) [**Vnguentum Rubeum.**] **Also for to make a rede oynement that is ryght good to dreye a wownde and to gadyr sownde esche and good and also for the kankyr and for a festryng sore.** Take a pownde of olde swynes grece and a quarte of jwse of plantayne and of Celondoyn. (…). (MEMT, 15th c. *WBMP* (MS Med. Misc. I), 312)

Only two writings[99], *Gilbertus Anglicus* (GA) and *Antidotarium Nicholai* (AntN) from the remedybook collection can boast of a high number of references to medicaments, 163 records (37% out of 442 records in remedy books) and 97 records (22%) respectively. This high proportion might be explained by the fact that these texts are 15th century translations of Latin originals and are often described as examples of a more learned layer of remedy book collections (Carrillo-Linares

98 As noted in chapter one, medieval recipes are characterised by a fairly regular structure. They are composed of (1) the heading, (2) list of ingredients, (3) advice on preparation and application of medicinal substances and (4) additional comments, usually focusing on the effectiveness of the recipe. The heading indicates the beginning of the recipe and, depending on the information included, can be divided into 4 types: (i) the statement of purpose that specifies the ailment or the medicament for which a given recipe is written: *For harness of þe splene, For to delyuer wynde and for þe colyk*, etc.; (ii) the name of the medicament (title): *Oximel, Pillule Aurere, Unguentum Populyoun, Yerapigra Galieni*, etc.; (iii) the name of the medicament and the statement of its purpose: *Syrop for þe feuer tercyane, A gude oyntment for alle feuers, Emplaster for þe gout*; (iv) expressions such as *Item, Another, Another for the same*, For the same, all of which were probably incorporated in order to avoid repetitions (Sylwanowicz 2015, Bator — Sylwanowicz 2017b).

99 *Antidotarium Nicholai* was written by Nicolaus Salernitanus, a 12th century teacher in the Medical School of Salerno. It is the most representative collection of recipes included in the *Remedies and materia medica* section of MEMT. Each recipe starts with a name of a medicine followed by an explanation of the origins of the name and by instructions of how a given medicine should be prepared and administered; cf. also Carillo-Linares (2005) or Pocuca — Stupar (2006). The latter text, *Gilbertus Anglicus*, is a 15th century translation of a Latin text written before 1250 by Gilbertus Anglicus – "England's first notable medical writer" (Getz 1991: xi). In this text, unlike in the *Antidotarium Nicholai*, recipes are part of longer texts, arranged in a head to foot order, and consisting of descriptions of sicknesses and their symptoms.

2005, Getz 1991, Pocuca — Stupar 2006). As for the remaining remedy book texts, the number of references to medicaments constitutes less than 10% of all records. For instance, in LeechB1, a collection of 142 recipes, there are only 15 (3% out of 442 records in remedy books) references to medical specifics. Similarly, in another collection of 293 recipes (REC) only 31 (7%) names of specifics are recorded.

As regards medieval surgical and specialised texts, they were mostly written by and for professionals and are generally characterised by technical instructional passages and a higher proportion of specialised terminology (cf. also Norri 1992, 1998, 2004; Sylwanowicz 2009, 2014a, 2015). As already noted in chapter two (cf. quotations about the requirements for a good surgeon) the authors of these texts assumed that the prospective readers/users of the medical collection would be experienced practitioners (or apprentices) with the same, shared medical knowledge, and there should be no need to repeat or explain what ought to be already known. For instance, in Guy de Chauliac's introduction to his *Chirurgia Magna* there is a passage instructing that a good surgeon should be familiar with and always keep with him at least five basic ointments:

(144) (…) he þat is a kyndely Cirurgian muste bere wiþ him.v. oynementis / þat is to wite. **Basilicon** to ripe wiþ. **Vnguentum apostolorum** to clense wiþ. **Vnguentum aureum** to regendre wiþ. **Unguentum album** to close wiþ. And **Dialtea** to liþe or souple wiþ. (Wallner, 1425 *GCM* (MS Cai 336/725), 9/13–19)

In addition, while going through these texts, one can observe that usually the authors only mention the name of the medicament and describe the way of its application, without any instruction on how to prepare it (145a). Alternatively, in some texts there are passages telling the reader that more detailed information on preparation and application is to be found in a separate section or chapter, often referred to as *þe antidotaria*[100] (145b).

(145) a. Þe toþer hole3, forsoþe, beyng bisyde it I cured wiþ cuttyng and with **puluer sine pare**. Euermore continuyng þe cure wiþ þe siryng in þe lefte side, and wiþ tentes als long as þay wolde entre in, and **þe emplastre Neyrbon** y-putte aboue, and **salus populi and vnguento Arabico**, (…). (Power, 1425 *AFS* (MS Sln 6), 34/22–27)
þilke discrasie þou schalt helpe wiþ coldynge þe lyme aboute þe wounde **with oile of rosis & vnguentum album, Rasis of ceruse**, (…). (Fleischhacker, a1400 *LSC1* (MS Ashm 1396), 57/4–6)
b. Þow schalt fynde a ful techinge of þese medicyns **in þe antidotarie** of þis book, þou schalt haue a ful techinge in þe antidotarie of mundificatiuis & cicatri3atiuis. (Fleischhacker, a1400 *LSC1* (MS Ashm 1396), 43/18–19)

100 The term *antidotaria* is explained in chapter two, section 2.6.

In þe þridde partie I haue putt an **antidotarie** of sirurgie wiþ watris, emplastris, poudris, oilis & oynementis, & oþere dyuers medicyns in general. (MEMT, 1475 *CHIR* (MS Wel 564), 1b)

The analysis of the material has also revealed that some terms are common to all texts, whereas some are peculiar to only one group of texts, i.e. some items are present either only in remedy books or surgical works or specialised treatises, and not elsewhere (cf. Figure 8 below).

Fig. 8: The relative normalized frequency (RNF per 100,000 words) of the names of specifics peculiar to all texts and to one type of text (absolute frequencies are in brackets)

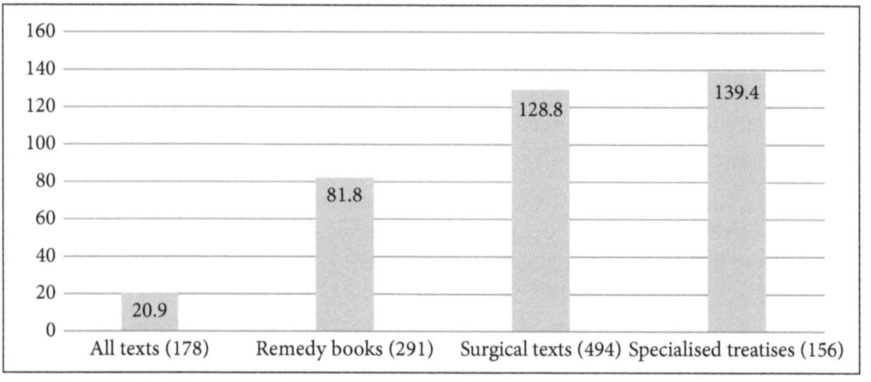

As seen in Figure 8, the group of terms recorded in all texts constitutes about a fifth of the total of 1119 items. These expressions include mostly medicaments for common ailments, e.g. preparations for: throat maladies (*gargarisma* and *diamoron*), eye disorders (*collyrie*), heaviness of the head (*diaspermaton*), or fevers (*diaprunis*); purgative medications (*benedicta, clyster, diapapaver, diagrydie, laxative, purgation*); ointments for boils, swellings, wounds or aches in joints and other parts of body (*agrippa, apostolicon* (= *ointment of apostles, unguentum apostolorum*), *basilicon, marciaton, unguentum aureum*).

Other recurrent examples constitute medicaments used to treat the disbalance of humours, e.g., *cold electuary, cold medicine, cold ointment, cold plaster, hot medicine, dry medicine, temperate medicine*, etc. There are also names of preparations with many uses, being either a basis for other mixtures, or used to treat a number of medical problems, e.g., *aqua vitae, oil of roses* (= *oleum rosaceum, oil roset*), *oil of violets* (= *oleum violaceum*), *oxymels, syrup of roses* (= *syrup rosat*), *syrup of violet, treacle* (= *theriac*), *water of roses* (*aqua rosarum, rose water*), etc.

These terms are not always evenly distributed in the three types of medical texts. For instance, *clyster*, *gargarisma* or *laxative* are more widespread in surgical works, whereas *fumigation* and *stufe*, both denoting therapeutic vapours and fumes, are more common in specialised treatises and remedy books. Among other words more frequently used in specialised texts and remedy books are names of various electuaries, e.g., *diacodion*, *diacuminum*, *dianisum*, *diarodon*, *electuarium de succo rosarum*, etc. Sometimes, the choice of words seems to have been determined by their form, i.e. more foreign-like forms are commonly found in learned texts. For instance, *unguentum apostolorum*, *unguentum viride* are much more frequent in surgical works, whereas their equivalents, *ointment of apostles*, *green ointment*, are evenly distributed in all three types of texts (for more on the use of foreign forms in the texts see the discussion further on in this section).

As regards the remaining 941 examples that are attested in only one variety of medical texts, there are also some differences in the use of terms. Similarly to the findings presented in Figure 7, the texts of a learned character (surgical works and specialised treatises) turn out to be a rich source of medical terminology, at least in the domain of the names for pharmaceuticals (650 vs. 291 items in remedy books). These learned texts are characterised by a much higher proportion of foreign and more technical vocabulary, e.g., *collyrium de plumbo*, *emplastrum de centaurea*, *oleum de spica*, *pilule de agarico*, *powder creoferoberon*, *salus populi*, *sief de plumbo*, *suppository provocative*, *tapsimel*, *trochisk de lactea*, *unguentum tetrapharmacum*, *virtus a Deo datum*, etc. Such expressions are also found in remedy books, but they are used sporadically and are often followed by their translations or explanations, cf.:

(146) (…) **oleum sambucinum**, þat ys, **oyle ymade of þe floeres of ellern** (…). (MEMT, 15th c. *AntN* (MS Ferguson 147), f. 9r)
To make vnguentum viridum. ffor to make **a grene oynement**. Take celendoyn, allelma, (…). (MEMT, 15th c. *WBMP* (MS Med. Misc. I), 312)

The expressions denoting the origin of the medicament, especially those referring to medical authorities, are also much more frequent in the learned sources (54 vs. 29 items in remedybooks), e.g., *cerote of Galien*, *liniment of Theodoric*, *medicine of Haly the Abbot*, *ointment of Master William Someris*, *syrup of Plateare*, *ointment of Four Masters*, *unguent of Master Dine*, have been found either in surgical or specialised texts but not in remedy books. Interestingly, in the latter writings, out of 29 items denoting the origin of the medicament 15 come from one text (AntN), e.g., *electuarium ducis*, *electuarium frigidum cophonis*, *katarticum imperiale*, *potio Santi Pauli*, *trifera saracenica*, etc.

A large number of terms are restricted to surgical texts, and these involve names of preparations used in the treatment of various injuries, skin disorders, swellings, growths or tumors, e.g., *burning medicine, cauterisative, corrosive water, incarnative, ointment ruptory*, etc. In the examined surgical sources, about 198 examples of preparations denoting therapeutic properties have been identified, which constitutes about 40% of all terms recorded in these texts. Although in specialised texts and remedy books there are also such terms, they are not as numerous as in surgical works (65 items in remedy books and 37 in specialised treatises, constituting 23% of all terms recorded in each category of texts) and they often denote less invasive preparations, i.e. soothing or moistening medicines (*comfortable drink, electuary comfortative, electuary humiditative, electuary moisting*), mixtures promoting tissue growth (*consolidative ointment*) or dissolving morbid matter (*plaster repercussive*), and some styptic preparations (*syrup constrictive, strictory medicine*).

Sometimes, references to medicaments depend on individual choices of the translators/compilers of foreign works. This is evident, for instance, in the two versions of Guy de Chauliac's text on *Anatomy* (GCA1 and GCA2)[101], where we find the following pairs[102]: *medicenes humectatiues* vs. *moystinge medecynes, medicenes of fractures* vs. *medecynes of broken bones, medicenes of dislocasions* vs. *medecynes of bones out of ioynte, medicenes caustices* vs. *dreieng medecynes, medicenes blode restrictiues* vs. *medecynes streynynge blood, doloure sedatiueȝ* vs. *medicynes of sorwes or akynges*, etc. Thus, the translator of the first version (GCA1) tends to adopt Latin forms, whereas in the latter version (GCA2) there are attempts to translate the terms into vernacular. Similarly, the two versions of Lanfranc's *Science of Cirurgie* (LSC1 and LSC2)[103] exhibit some differences in the way the references to medicaments are presented. These involve, for instance:

(i) the etymology of the selected word, e.g., *enoynture* (OF) vs. *vncture* (L), *vnguento* (AN < L) *fusco* vs. *oygnement* (OF) *fusco*;
(ii) the choice of structural patterns (i.e. either Germanic (adj + noun), the Latin/French (noun + adj.) noun modification pattern, or the use of *of*-phrases),

101 A detailed description of these two manucripts is to be found in chapter three.
102 In each pair the first example comes from GCA1, whereas the second from GCA2. The examples listed here retain original pronunciation, as found in the text editions.
103 LSC1 stands for MS Bodleian Ashmole 1396, ff. 2v-29v and is dated back to about 1400, whereas LSC2 is a collection of texts found in the British Library, Additional 12056, dated back to about 1450 (cf. MED). In the above discussion, the first example in the list of names comes from LSC1, whereas the second from LSC2.

e.g., *plastre maturatijf* vs. *maturatyff plastre, oile of laurine* vs. *oyle lauryne, decoccioun epithimum* vs. *decoccioun of Epytemum, oile of rue* vs. *Oyle rewe*;

(iii) the choice of a wordform, e.g., *consolidaciouns* (noun) vs. *consolidatyfes* (noun < adj.), *perfiȝt mundificatif* (noun < adj.) vs. *perfyte mundificacioun* (noun);

(iv) spelling, e.g., *oile enfancinum* (erroneous spelling of L *omphancinum*, cf. MED, *omfacinum* n.) vs. *oyle Omfancinum*.

These differences reveal that the translators were often inconsistent in the way they presented technical vocabularies.

A group of names are recorded in the texts of a single writer. For instance, in the treatise on eye diseases and injuries by Benvenutus Grassus[104] (BG), we find references to some pills (*pillule Iherosolimitane, pillule Benvenuci*), powders (*Nabateans' powder, pulvis Nabatinus, pulvis Alexandrini, pulvis benedictus*), ointments (*colerium Alexandrinum, colerium Iherosolimitanum, ointment of alabaster, unguentum alabastri, unguentum subtile*), an electuary (*diolibanum Salernitanum*), a plaster (*emplastrum laudabile*), and some cleansing medicine for the eyes (*clarificacio oculorum*). It is possible that most of these medicaments were compounded by Grassus himself, as we find passages where he stresses the fact of being the author of a preparation, cf.:

(147) (…) yt may be curyd with **my colery that ys clepyd colerium Iherosolimitanum** that ys mayd yn thyse wyse: Take tutie (…). (MEMT, 1474–1499 *BG* (MS Hunter V.8.6), 59)

(…) ley on the ey **my plaster clepyd emplastrum laudabile** (…) yt swagyth the bolnyng, it settyth the eye fyxe yn hys place, it lesseth the payn, and refreshyth the syght; and **for thies causes I cal it laudable**, that ys worthy to be praysed. (MEMT, 1474–1499 *BG* (MS Hunter V.8.6), 75)

104 From the English translation of *De probatissima arte oculorum*, a treatise on eye disorders, we learn that its author was "A grete phylosopher and a profunde phycycyane clepid Benuonucius Grapheus, after the sentence of þe olde auctors of phelozophie and of phisyk whiche he had radde, and after hys propre experyence the wych he had by long contynuance of his owne practik yn dyuerse parties of the world, boyth yn hote regyons and colde, by influence and help of goddys grace, compilyd and made a boke of the sekenes of eyon and of her curys: and entitled thys boke and clepid it Deus oculorum." (MEMT, 1474–1499 *BG* (MS Hunter V.8.6), 49). The text examined for the present study is one of the two surviving Middle English versions of the original writing, edited by Eldredge (1996). For more on Benvenutus Grassus and his works see: Eldredge (1998, 1999), Palmer (2006), Garcia — Fernández-Corugedo (2011). There is also a doctoral dissertation on the diachronic evolution of the nomenclature of ophthalmology in English medical language by Esteve Ramos (2008).

And þan put yn hys ey at morn and euyn of **my powder callyd puluis nabetus** tyl the eye be clere sufficyently. (MEMT, 1474–1499 *BG* (MS Hunter V.8.6), 76)
(…) lete hym resceyue of **our electuarye clepyd dyaolibanum Salernitanum** tyl he be hole. (MEMT, 1474–1499 *BG* (MS Hunter V.8.6), 68)

In the surgical treatises of John Arderne we find names not used elsewhere, e.g., *emplaster of Nerbon* (in short *Nerbon*), *powder creoferoberon, powder sine pari, salus populi, valence of scabious, valence of wormwood.* Some of them are not mere translations or adoptions of Latin originals, but names of the medicaments introduced by the surgeon himself (*emplaster of Nerbon, sine pari*). Thus, English authors of medical texts did not rely solely on other sources and medical authorities but used their own experience in the healing practice.

As regards the etymology of the terms under discussion, they can be divided into three main groups: (i) Romance, (ii) Germanic, and (iii) hybrid formations. The first group consists of the names that were imported into English from French or Latin. These forms have been included in one category labeled as Romance because it is not always possible to determine the exact provenance of the terms (cf. Wallner 1969, Strang 1970, Norri 1992, 2004, 2016). This is especially true of "those words which in French are not popular survivals of spoken Latin words, but are later borrowings from literary Latin." (Jespersen 1972: 107, after Norri 1992: 112). We can find here forms that had been recorded already in Old English medical writings[105], e.g., *oxymel* 'a medicinal potion made of honey and vinegar' which was recorded in Old English sources as *oxumel* alongside its translations: *suþerne læcedom* or *suþeren eceþ drenc*; *oil of roses* recorded as *ȝerosode ele* or *ele ro.*, and *tiriac* 'an antidote against poisons' as *tiriaca.* The remaining examples of the Romance terms are forms that first occurred in the Middle English writings.

The Germanic group is represented by forms that had a medical sense already in Old English (*bath*), items that gained medical sense in Middle English (*cleanser, dwale, sape*), or Middle English translations of foreign terms, e.g., *burning water* < L *aqua ardent, chewing* < L *masticatio, dry bath* < L *balneum siccum, strong water,* < L *aqua fortis, washing* < L *lavamentum, water ironed* < L *aqua ferrata, water of ashes* < L *aqua cineris.*

The last group, hybrid formations, consists of derivatives with French or Latin roots and the English suffix *-ing*, e.g., *defending, frotting, straining*, and compounds or phrases exhibiting the following patterns: a native form + loan form

105 Cf. the earliest English medical writings edited by Cockayne (1864–1866) and Vriend (1984).

(*bath strictory, black entrete, burning medicine, drink alterative, red ointment, water ardent*, etc.), and a loan form + a native form (*alum water, emplaster drying, medicine riping, valence of wormwood*, etc.). The forms used in hybrids can be divided into semantic groups. The Germanic element is represented by nouns denoting ingredients as in *plaster of leek, powder of dill, syrup of wormwood*, and dosage forms as in *ball of aloes, drink alterative, water ardent*, where the forms with *water* constitute one third of all collected hybrids. Other groups of Germanic items constitute adjectives alluding to humoral theory (*cold medicine, hot electuary, dry syrup*), indicating the colour of the medicaments (*black ointment, green entrete, red powder, white collyrie*), or their curative properties (burning *medicine, biting suppository, sharp medicine*). As regards a Romance element in the hybrid formations, these are names of dosage forms (e.g. *cold pilule, cold syrup, hot plaster, oil of hocks, red ointment, powder of barley*), names of specifics (e.g. *cold diuretic, collyrie of lede, valence of wormwood*), and a general term for medical preparations (e.g. *hot medicine, strong medicine*, etc.). There are also names of ingredients (e.g. *water of celidony, water of plantain, water of tartar*, etc.) and adjectives indicating propeties of medicaments (e.g. *comfortable drink, corrosive water, drink alterative*, etc.). The ratio of the occurrence the terms of different origin that have been identified in the examined texts is presented in Figure 9 below.

Fig. 9: The percentage of the occurrences of forms of different origin (Romance, Germanic, hybrid forms)

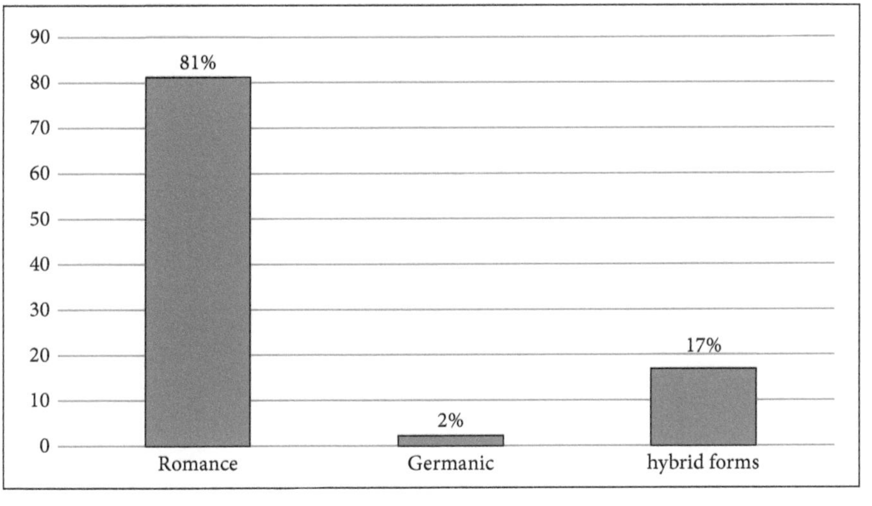

The data clearly shows that names of Romance origin were predominant and they seem to confirm a general tendency in the English medical language to adopt foreign forms. This large number of foreign terms is not unexpected as most Middle English medical texts were translated from or derived from Latin or French treatises. Hybrid forms and Germanic words, on the other hand, illustrate modest attempts at vernacularization of English medical terminology, at least in the domain of the names of medicaments.

A closer examination of the distribution of the forms of different origin in the three text types reveals the same pattern (cf. Figure 10 below). Thus, in each group of texts Romance words are prevalent, followed by hybrid formations and the names of Germanic origin. There are, however, some differences which again indicate that the choice of forms depended largely on the level of the text or on its compiler. As Figure 10 shows, the proportion of the Romance forms in remedy-books, surgical works and specialised treatises is not equal (cf. RNF: 94.8, 126.3 and 164.6 respectively). These results clearly demonstrate that there was a marked preference for foreign forms in the writings representing a more learned register.

Fig. 10: The relative normalized frequency (RNF per 100,000 words) of the forms of different origin in three types of medical texts

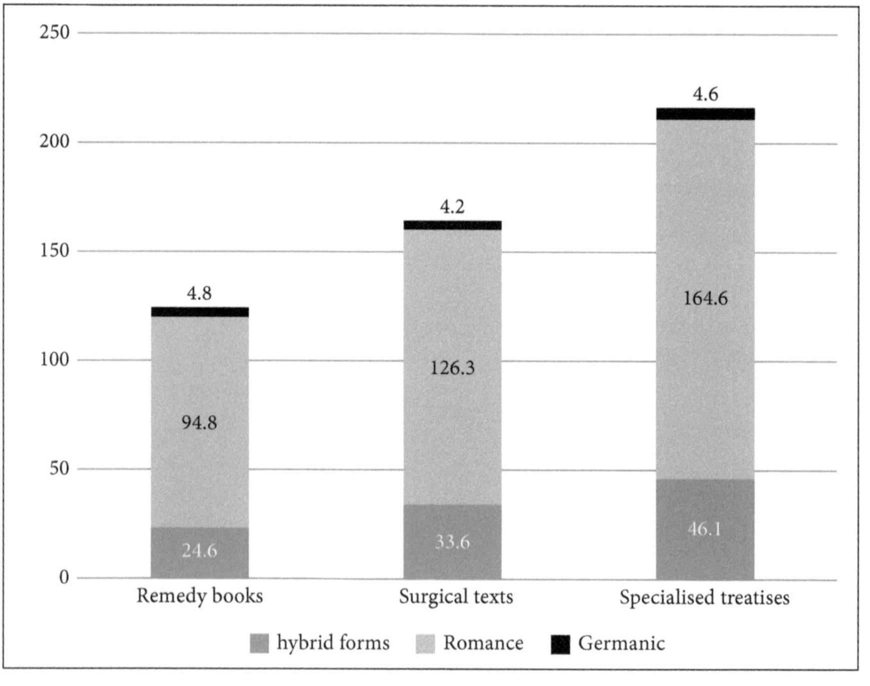

The tendency to use foreign forms over hybrids or native items is evident in each text categorised as surgical and specialised. A thorough reading of these texts and the analysis of the distribution of forms of different origin has revealed that in each writing the number of references to medicaments is fairly high, and the Romance forms constitute about 90–97% of all the recorded names. For instance, in Lanfranc's writings (LSC1/LSC2) the proportion between Romance, Germanic and hybrid forms is 147/1/9 respectively, in Arderne's text (AFS) 94/1/6, in Guy de Chauliac's treatise on ulcers (GCU) 86/2/10, and in his treatise on wounds (GCW) 66/0/2. As regards specialised texts, the proportions are similar, e.g., 70/0/10 (SW2), 33/0/4 (SW1), 31/0/1 (BG).

In the remedy books, the distribution of examined names is not equally proportional in each text. As indicated earlier in this section, the highest number of all names has been recorded in two texts (AntN and GA). In the first text, all references to medicaments (97 items) are of Romance origin, and in the latter they constitute about 70% (110 out of 163). As regards the remaining texts, references to medicaments are sporadic. Although foreign forms still prevail in these texts, e.g., 10/0/3 (JBurg), 22/0/0 (CExp), 22/0/6 (WBMP), 6/0/1 (LDM), etc., the results cannot be treated as indicators of a preference for foreign forms in remedy book collections. In addition, most of the foreign forms recorded in remedy books are references to medicaments present in almost all medical texts examined for the present study[106], e.g., *comfortatives* (Rem.: 10, Surg.: 5, Spec.: 2), *fumigation* (Rem.: 23, Surg.: 4, Spec.: 24), *hierapigra* (Rem.: 5, Surg.: 2, Spec.: 3), *laxatives* (Rem.: 16, Surg.: 19, Spec.: 2), *oleum rosaceum* (Rem.: 10, Surg.: 18, Spec.: 3), *syrup rosate* (Rem.: 4, Surg.: 3, Spec.: 4), *treacle* (Rem.: 7, Surg.: 8, Spec.: 12), *unguentum albumum* (Rem.: 6, Surg.: 10, Spec.: 4), *unguentum viridum* (Rem.: 5, Surg.: 19, Spec.: 4), etc. The circulation of these particular specifics in a variety of medical texts suggests that they denoted fairly well-known medicaments, and it is likely that despite their foreign form some of them were understood by not very experienced medical practitioners, or even lay users of medical books.

The adoptions of foreign forms and new coinages resulted in a very large number of names of medicaments. In many cases, the same preparation was referred to by a variety of forms, e.g., *red salve, red ointment, unguentum rubeum* (cf. also examples in section 5.3.1). This terminological maze reflected the fact that the compilers or translators of medical texts often varied in renderring words of foreign origin (cf. the earlier discussion of the discrepancies in the choice of words

106 The numbers are absolute frequencies of the terms in each collection of texts. Rem. = Remedy books, Surg. = Surgical texts, Spec. = Specialised treatises.

in the English versions of works attributed to Guy de Chauliac and Lanfranc). In addition, the authors of medical manuals often differed in naming the same medicament, which often might have led to either confusion or incorrect use of these terms. This situation is described in the following fragment from Lanfranc's *Sciencie of Cirurgie*:

(148) It þinkiþ bi þe maner of speche þat medicyns þat ben seid in þis chapitre ben al oon, but þer is miche difference bitwixe / ffor of summen alle þei ben clepid consolidatiuis. But aggregatiue & consolidatiue ben al oon / And regeneratiue, & incarnatiue, & facientes carnem nasci, ben oon to seie; & þer is greet difference bitwixe hem þat ben forseid & þese (…); neþeles alle þeses names ben not propirly take of alle auctoris / But oon herof is taken for anoþer ofte tyme / But for to seie þe soþe, a medicin þat is clepid aggregatum or conglutinatum, & A. in diuers placis taketh diuersli þese names of medicyns: & I suppose þat it were for defaute of men þat translatid þe science. (Fleischhacker, a1400 *LSC1* (MS Ashm 1396), 342/18–29)

The above passage concentrates on a number of references to closing medicines (*aggregative, consolidative, incarnative, regenerative*) and to a slight difference between them. From the later fragments we learn that *aggregatiues* and *consolidatiues* are names of preparations that close wounds through drying the wound, whereas *regeneratiue* and *incarnatiue* mixtures promote the growth of tissue or flesh. The author of the text directs our attention to the fact that these differences seem to have been ignored in the writings of Avicenna (in the text referred to as A.). This, however, is probably not the fault of the author of the text but of "men þat translatid þe science" (Fleischhacker, a1400 *LSC1* (MS Ashm 1396), 342/29).

Based on the above, it is clear that renderring medical texts posed quite a challenge to the translators. Nevertheless, the examination of the texts has shown that their compilers tried to avoid misinterpretations and used a variety of techniques that might have facilitated the understanding of new or difficult terms.

One way of explaining new terms was the use of repetitive word pairs or binomials[107], i.e. two words that belong to the same grammatical category, and are semantically related (Kopaczyk — Sauer 2017: 3). These expressions are formed mostly

107 The term *repetitive word pairs* was proposed by Koskenniemi (1968). To alternative terms used in literature belong, among others, tautological pairs (Leisi 1947), conjoined phrases (Tiersma 1999), word pairs (Tani 2010), paired opposites (Cummings 1980), etc. The majority of works prefer the term *binomial*, which is not as restrictive as previous terms (cf. Kopaczyk — Sauer 2017: 8). The term was introduced by Malkiel (1959) and it was used in a number of other studies, e.g., Gustafsson (1975), Kopaczyk (2009, 2013), (Mollin 2014), etc. For a detailed account of binomials in the history of English see Kopaczyk — Sauer (2017).

with the use of the connective forms, *and* and *or.* The present study is concentrated on structures in which the components are "near-synonyms", i.e. they "refer to the same thing, though perhaps seen from a slightly different angle" (Koskenniemi 1968: 91). The examples found in the examined material consist of constructions in which the Romance element is usually used side by side with the native element that served as an interpretation of a less familiar foreign form, cf.:

(149) (…) with **medycines resoluyng and rypyng** and þe postumes (…). (MEMT, 1500 LChP (MS Wel 397), 85)
The medesynes caterysatif and brennyng to fester and cankr shall be said in þe ende (…). (MEMT, 1500 LChP (MS Wel 397), 88)

Sometimes, the instances of two Romance elements were linked together, which may imply that one of these expressions was a commonly recognised form in English, cf.:

(150) Galyen seith that **purgaciouns** and **vomytes** shulde be take but seldom and for gret nede. (MEMT, 15th c. GovH (MS Sln 989), f. 13v)
And suche **stufes** or **fumigacions** shullen be (…). (Getz, a1475 *GA* (MS Wel 537), 66/13)

This explicatory technique was frequently applied in enhancing the understanding of the names of sicknesses (Norri 1992, Sylwanowicz 2014a) or body parts (Norri 1998). As regards the names of medicaments, only few examples show the use of this technique.

To more common explicatory phrases belong interpolations and explanations, especially of the *þat is (clepid)* type, or its Latin counterpart *id est (.i.).* One group consists of examples where the foreign form follows or precedes a more familiar equivalent, cf.:

(151) (…) and afterwards mak **oile of þe asshe** *þat is yclepid* **fraxinus** (MEMT, 1450–1475 *MedCh* (MS Add 34111), 125)
a medycyne caustyk - *þat is to sigge*, **brennynge** (Fleischhacker, a1450 *LSC2* (MS Add 12056), 93/38)
lauamenteȝ.*i.* **wasshyngȝ** (Wallner, 1425 *GCU* (MS NY 12), 81/2)
Oxirodinum.*i.* **oile of rosis with a litel acete** (Wallner, 1425 *GCW* (MS NY 12), 51/17)
a medecene liptomer.*i.* **diaforetic** (Wallner, 1425 *GCW* (MS NY 12), 83/22)
vnguento viridi, *i.* **grene oyntment of lanfrank** (Power, 1425 *AFS* (MS Sln 6), 54/4)
oleum plumby, *i.* **oyle of lede** (MEMT, 1475 QE (MS Sln 73), 193)

Sometimes, a foreign term is not translated but only introduced by a general term (e.g. *medicine*), or a name of dosage form (e.g. *plaster, ointment*), cf.:

(152) (…) wiþ **a medicyn** *þat is clepid* **trociscus de turbit**
(Fleischhacker, a1400 *LSC1* (MS Ashm 1396), 200/11–12)
Medcyn *þat is called* **Gratia Dei** (MEMT, 1440 *LDM* (MS Thornton A.5.2), 68)
Syrop *þat es called* **þe Rose**. [(MEMT, 1440 *LDM* (MS Thornton A.5.2), 60)
(…) an **enplayst~** *that is clepid* **enpleyst~ capitall of mayster anselme of jene**
(MEMT, c 1450 *LeechB1* (MS Med-L 136), 44)
And on the stepe of the wonde there the sore was ley on an **oynement** callyd **vnguentum subtile**. (MEMT, 1474–1499 *BG* (MS Hunter V.8.6), 79)

In addition to the above examples, there are passages where the term is not translated but followed by a definition, providing information on the use and application, or the main ingredients the relevant mixture is composed of, cf.:

(153) 3yve him a **cologoge,** *þat is to sey,* **a medicyn þat may clense him and purge him of coler** (…). (Getz, a1475 *GA* (MS Wel 537), 35/14–15)
And let him ete diapenidion with **ptisane. (Ptisane is watir þat barliche is soden yn.**) (Getz, a1475 *GA* (MS Wel 537), 108/2)

Providing the explanations of the origin of the term is another method of presenting foreign forms. Usually, a Latin expression is given first and then it is followed by an explanation as to why a given medicament is so called, cf.:

(154) **DIAMORON.**Yt haþe his name for yt ys made of beryes. (MEMT, 15th c. *AntN* (MS Ferguson 147), f. 10r)
IGIA GRECA. Igia, þat ys to sey, a sauour. **Greca,** of þe peple of grekes furste yt was yfounde. (MEMT, 15th c. *AntN* (MS Ferguson 147), f. 27r)
Puluis sine pari, or **french Poudre sanȝ pere,** is made þus: Recipe (…). **Þis poudre** is seid **"without pere" ffor it haþe no pere in wirchyng;** (Power, 1425 *AFS* (MS Sln 6), 86/23, 32)

The examples above and the examination of the texts have shown that it was not always necessary to fill English lexicon with foreign, especially Latin technical terminology. For instance, instead of *unguentum viridum* or *albumum*, one could have used *green salve* or *white salve.* Similarly, *medicines infrigidatif/mundificative/caustic* could have been renderred as *kelynge/clensynge/brennynge medicines*, where only the term *medicine* is a foreign adoption. The question is, what motivated the compilers to use foreign instead of already known forms.

One of the possible explanations is that compilers may have used the foreign form for reasons of style or prestige (cf. Pahta 2004). Thus, the more learned text the more sophisticated and foreign forms. This is confirmed by the discussion of Figure 10, which shows the distribution of foreign forms in the three types of texts. Thus, the more learned text the more foreign or "sophisticated" forms are present. Another possible explanation is that some foreign terms are more precise, cf.:

(155) Here ye shal vndrestande þat **þere is difference bitwyne corrosifes** and **vlceratifz**. Corrosifes, been þay hote or colde, þay muste neede be drie; and þay muste be litel in quantite whenne þay be put on the or on þe flessh. But vlceratifz matieres been sum what mightier þenne þe corrosifz, ffor þay þat been vlceratif been ordenned to pershe þe skyn þe whiche [{is{] euer harder þenne þe flessh. For |as the corrosife fretith þe flessh, right so vlceratife fretith the skynne; (MEMT, 15th c. *RupQ* (MS Ferguson 205), 176)

According to the above, the two forms (*corrosives* and *ulceratives*) refer to medicines that might be explained as some sort of burning medicines (ME *brennynge medecyne*). However, *corrosives* were medicines that 'destroyed organic tissue', whereas *ulceratives* were stronger in effect as they were 'breaking skin and causing ulceration' (cf. also DMVE, *corrosive medicne* n. and *ulcerative medicine* n.). Hence the tendency to use foreign terms that are more accurate in meaning than many Middle English formations.

5.5 Summary

The group of terms denoting specifics is definitely most numerous in terms of references to medical preparations (at least 1646 instances). Hence, the collected material has been divided into two large categories on the basis of the word formation structure, i.e. (1) simplex terms and derivatives and (2) compounds and phrases. The former consists of 384 instances, and the latter of 1262.

Within each category (i.e. simplex terms and derivatives, and compounds and phrases), the terms have been further divided into five semantic groups:

(i) names indicating the main ingredients (of plant, animal and mineral origin);
(ii) names indicating the origin of the medicament, i.e. names that indicate medical authorities, historical figures, religious/divine authorities, place of origin;
(iii) names indicating a body part or a medical condition to be cured;
(iv) names indicating therapeutic methods (only simplex forms and derivatives);
(v) names indicating the properties of medicaments.

The first and the last group can boast of the highest number of references to medicaments. The former consists of 717 instances (43%) and the latter of 669 instances (41%). They are followed by a group of names indicating the origin of the medicament, with 160 instances (10%). The remaining two categories (ii and iv) are marginally represented and altogether consist of 34 items (about 2%).

There is also a number of terms, 66 instances (4%), that do not fit in any of the above categories, and hence they are discussed as miscellaneous names.

The examination of the distribution of the names of medical preparations in the three types of medical writings has revealed that the the texts representing learned register (surgical works and specialised treatises) have a much higher proportion of terms, especially those of a more technical character than remedy books (cf. Figure 7). Similar contrast is seen in the distribution of forms of different etymologies. Although forms of Romance origin prevail in all text-types (cf. Figure 10), these forms seem to be evenly distributed in all writings belonging to the group of learned texts, whereas in remedy books the use of such terms seems to be haphazard. As regards the use of various techniques used to explain foreign adoptions (e.g. repetitive word pairs, *that is (clepid)* formulas, information on differences between the terms or on their origin), such examples are also more common in texts representing the learned layer.

Conclusions

The present study aimed at giving a comprehensive critical review of Middle English names of medical preparations found in the available medical works (remedy books, surgical texts and specialised treatises) produced in the 14th–15th centuries, and in a number of dictionaries. Particular attention has been paid to the origin of the terms, their structure, and their distribution and presentation in texts representing different traditions of medical writing.

The lexical field pertaining to the concept of medical preparations consists of at least 1695 references to medicaments (cf. also Table 11 below), of which the majority constitute items of Romance origin (77%). The remainig group of terms includes hybrid formations (17%), Germanic forms (5%), and terms of unknown origin (less than 1%). Although the majority of the collected expressions entered the medical lexicon of English in the 14th–15th centuries, some of them (at least 10 examples, 5 of Germanic and 5 of Romance provenance) had already been used in Old English medical writings.

Tab. 11: The number of Middle English references to medical preparations in the analysed material

	General terms denoting medical preparations		Terms denoting dosage forms		Terms denoting specifics			
	Germanic	Romance	Germanic	Romance	Germanic	Romance	Hybrids	Unknown
Simplex terms and derivatives	3	6	4	36	21	357	3	3
Compounds and phrases	-	-	-	-	56	909	297	-

In order to facilitate the examination of the terms, they have been divided into three major categories: (i) general terms denoting medical preparations, (ii) terms denoting dosage forms, and (iii) terms denoting specifics. Within each category they have been further subdivided into a number of groups. Thus, general terms denoting medical preparations have been divided according to their origin (Germanic and Romance terms). The next category of terms has been devised on the basis of their meaning: general terms denoting semisolid, solid and liquid preparations. The last and the largest group of words and expressions, i.e. names denoting specifics, has been discussed as simplex terms and derivatives, and compounds and phrases. The names of specifics have been further divided into five semantic groups: (i) names indicating the main ingredient(s), (ii) names indicating the origin (e.g. authors or place) of the preparation, (iii) names indicating body parts or medical condition, (iv) names denoting therapeutic methods, and (v) names indicating the properties of the preparations. In addition, a number of terms that do not fit in any of the five categories have been discussed in separate sections as miscellaneous forms. The diverse division of the terms allows one to observe the rivalry between items related by meaning or form but of different etymology. Also, it is possible to scrutinize the word formation patterns that prevailed in the formation of terms. In addition, the division into semantic groups (cf. names of specifics in chapter five) provides an insight into the traditions lying behind the preparation of pharmaceutical mixtures in Medieval England.

As noted earlier in this section, the largest group of references to medical preparations consists of terms of French or Latin provenance (1308 items). They form a part of the central and common medical vocabulary, e.g., *electuary*, *emplaster*, *medicine*, *ointment*, *plaster*, *powder*, *syrup*, all of which are very frequent in all types of medical writings. Some of these forms are also commonly used as head nouns in compounds and phrases (e.g. about 178 instances with *medicine*, 72 with *powder*, 62 with *emplaster*, 55 with *plaster*, 45 with *syrup*, 42 with *ointment*, cf. Appendix B). Apart from common terms, adoptions of Romance origin include also less common forms, often being of a more technical character, e.g., *antidotum ymagogum*, *encatisma*, *extinguentia*, *conglutinativum*, *philantropos*, *pulvis consolidativus*, *theodoricon expericito laxativa*, etc. (cf. also Appendix A and B).

The forms of English origin are not as numerous as those of Romance provenance (84 instances, cf. also Table 11 above). Although some of these terms (e.g. *bath*, *cleansing*, *drink*, *salve*, *water*) had already been used in Old English medical writings, their use and distribution in the examined Middle English writings is marginal. This is partly due to the fact that each of these forms had to compete with their numerous foreign counterparts. For instance, in the group of 11 salve-like preparations, the noun *salve* was the only Germanic form (cf. also the number of occurrences of Fr. *ointment* (378 records) vs. Gmc *salve* (23 records), Table 4 in chapter four). The only English noun, which can boast of a relatively high frequency of use is *water*. Although it has only 11 records as a single term, it has been recorded as a head noun in 152 compounds and phrases (cf. Appendix B). In addition, native forms seem to have been restricted to remedy book texts, which represent an older tradition of medical writing and are often regarded as collections of texts of a less learned character. The examination of all three text-types has also revealed that native forms are mostly documented in explicatory phrases. Thus, native forms were not considered as highly technical terms and their main function was to facilitate the understanding of probably more prestigious but not-yet-familiar terms.

Another category of terms to be considered from the etymological point of view constitute hybrid formations. They are fairly well represented (about 300 instances) and are found in the group of names denoting specifics. There are only three derivatives with the French or Latin root and the English suffix *-ing*, e.g., *defending, frotting, straining*. The remaining instances are recorded in the group of compounds and phrases. They exhibit the following patterns: a native form + a loan form (*bath strictory, black entrete, burning medicine, drink alterative, red ointment, water ardent*, etc.), and a loan form + a native form (*alum water, emplaster drying, medicine riping, valence of wormwood*, etc.).

The Germanic element is mostly represented by nouns denoting ingredients, adjectives alluding to humoral theory, indicating the colour of the medicaments, or their curative properties. References to dosage forms are rather infrequent (e.g. *salve* is found in only 3 expressions, *drink* in 6, and *ball* in 5; cf. Appendix B), the only exception being the already mentioned noun *water*.

The Romance element, in contrast, apart from nouns denoting ingredients (e.g. *water of celidony, water of plantain, water of tartar*, etc.) and adjectives indicating propeties of medicaments (e.g. *comfortable drink, corrosive water, drink alterative*, etc.), is represented by a high number of names denoting dosage forms (e.g. *cold pilule, cold syrup, hot plaster, oil of hocks, red ointment, powder of barley*, etc.), names of specifics (e.g. *cold diuretic, collyrie of lede, valence of wormwood*, etc.), and the use of a general term for medical preparations as a head noun (e.g. *hot medicine, strong medicine*, etc.).

A large number of terms of foreign origin directs our attention to the fact that finding adequate English words or expressions for the names of medicaments may have posed some sort of a challenge to the translators/compilers of the medical texts. Although, as pointed out earlier, occasionally native expressions were used, copyists usually transferred French or Latin terms that, in turn, might have been unfamiliar to the users of the manuals. However, a study of the texts has revealed that a number of techniques were employed to facilitate the understanding of the terms. A common explicatory technique was the use of repetitive word pairs, usually combined with connectives *and/or, þat is (clepid)* or its Latin counterpart *id est* (*.i.*). In these constructions, the explanatory item is either a Germanic form (e.g. *salues* and *entretis, lauamenteȝ*.i. *wasshyngȝ*), or an already familiar Romance element (e.g. *purgaciouns* and *vomytes, a medicyn* þat is clepid *trociscus de turbit*). Another way to explain less known forms was to comment on their origin and/or provide information on what sort of ailments might be cured with a preparation referred to by a given name. Etymological explanations are more common in the writings of a learned character, and are often provided by the authors of the medicaments (e.g. John Arderne's explanations for *nerbon* or *puluis sine pari*).

If we consider the structure of the examined forms, simplex terms and derivatives constitute only one third of the total inventory of 1695 items. They consist of general terms denoting medical preparations, terms denoting dosage forms and specifics. The majority of these terms constitute adoptions of Romance terms (cf. Table 11). Within this group, many instances are:

(i) nouns with the Latin prefix *dia-* 'made of' combined with items denoting the main ingredient of the preparation (e.g. *diacastoreum*, *diapapaver*, *diasene*, etc.),
(ii) agent nouns with the Latin suffix *-ive* (e.g. *extractive*, *frigidative*, *mundificative*, *preservative*, *purgative*, etc.), and
(iii) agent nouns ending in *-er* (e.g. *enfreider*, *infreider*, *leptomer*).

The third group constitute either adoptions of French forms (e.g. *comforter* < OF *conforteur*, AN *confortere*, *defender* < OF *defendeor*, MF *defendeur*) or combinations of ME verb and suffix *-er*, e.g. *blisterer* (*blister* 'to cause blistering' < OF n. *blestre* + *-er*). In addition, there are also fifteen words of Germanic origin which end in the suffix *-er* (e.g. *breaker*, *keeler*, *riper*). Another English suffix (*-ing*) is employed in only five instances, of which three are hybrid formations (*defending*, *frotting*, *straining*), and two native formations (*fnesing*, *helping*).

As regards compounds and phrases, which are prevalent in the analysed lexical field, they are found only in the group of names denoting specifics. These forms are either direct loans from French or Latin, or Middle English translations of foreign terms. As a result, the following major structural patterns can be distinguished (listed in order of their frequency):

(i) combinations in which the head noun is followed by *of*-phrases (e.g. *emplaster of plantain*, *ointment of myrtles*, *pilule of rhubarb*, etc.),
(ii) combinations in which the head noun is followed by a modifier, i.e. so called French/Latin pattern (e.g. *medicine diaphoretic*, *plaster restrictive*, *water ardent*, etc.),
(iii) combinations in which the head noun is preceded by a modifier, i.e. so called Germanic model (*breaking ointment*, *drying emplaster*, *solutive medicine*, etc.),
(iv) combinations in which the head noun is followed by *de*-phrases (e.g. *collyrium de plumbo*, *sief de plumbo*, *treacle de boys*, etc.), and

(v) combinations with the *s*-genitive (e.g. *Galen's powder, King's ointment, Master Dine's powder*, etc.).

Apart from linguistic issues, the analysis of the names of medical preparations provides also an insight into the pharmaceutical practice in Medieval England. A large number of names denoting the main ingredient (of plant, animal, or mineral origin) reveal a great reliance on the "gifts" of Mother Nature. References to medical authorities equip us with information on classical and contemporary practitioners that were influential in the Middle Ages. Similarly, terms with the adjectives *cold, hot* or *dry* (e.g. *cold electuary, hot ointment, dry syrup*), reflect the importance of the principles of humoral theory in medieval medical practice. Last but not least, many names denoting healing properties of the medicament depict typical medical problems (especially various wounds and other injuries) and, somehow, turn our attention to the importance of the work of surgeons.

The present work proves that, contrary to a number of earlier studies (e.g. Knowles 1997, Schäfer 1989), Middle English was not deficient in scientific terms. Although the terminology was not uniform and a large number of references or variant forms to the same medicament made the English lexicon of pharmaceutical products some sort of "a terminological labirynth" (Norri 2016: 2), the 14th and especially 15th century laid solid foundations for the development of English scientific vocabularies, at least in the domain of medicine.

References

(a) Dictionaries

Anglo-Norman Dictionary (*AND*). 2001. Online edition available at http://www.anglo-norman.net (date of access: June 2016 – September 2017).

Ayto, John. 1990. *Bloomsbury Dictionary of Word Origins*. London: Bloomsbury.

Bosworth, Joseph — T. Northcote Toller. 1898. *An Anglo-Saxon Dictionary.* Online edition available at www.bosworthtoller.com (date of access: June 2015 – November 2017).

Dictionary of Medieval Latin from British Sources (*DMLBS*). 2013. Online edition available at http://www.dmlbs.ox.ac.uk (date of access: June 2015 – November 2017).

diPaolo Healey, Antonette — Dorothy Haines — Joan Holland — David McDougall — Ian McDougall (eds.). 2008. *Dictionary of Old English: A to G*, with electronic version for Windows developed by Xin Xiang. Toronto: Dictionary of Old English Project, on CD-ROM.

Dorland's Medical Dictionary (*DMD*). 2012. Philadelphia: Elsevier. Online edition, available at https://dorlandsonline.com/dorland/dictionary (date of access: June 2015 – November 2017).

Historical Thesaurus of English. Oxford University Press: online edition, available at www.oed.com/thesaurus (date of access: June 2015 – September 2017).

McSparran, Frances (ed.). *The Middle English Compendium: Middle English Dictionary, HyperBibliography, and Corpus of Middle English Prose and Verse.* http://ets.umdl.umich.edu/m/mec/. Ann Arbor: Humanities Text Initiative – University of Michigan, (date of access: June 2015 – September 2017).

Norri, Juhani. 2016. *Dictionary of Medical Vocabulary in English, 1375–1550.* New York: Ashgate.

Oxford English Dictionary. Oxford University Press: online edition, available at http://oed.com (date of access: June 2015 – September 2017).

Roberts, Jane — Christian Kay — Jane Roberts — Lynne Grundy (eds.). 2000. *A Thesaurus of Old English* (TOE). London: King's College London Centre for Late Antique and Medieval Studies.

(b) Text corpus sources

Alonso Almeida, Francisco (ed.). 2014. *A Middle English Medical Remedy Book from Glasgow University Library MS Hunter 185*. (*Middle English Texts* 50). Heidelberg: Universitätsverlag Winter.

Cockayne, Oswald (ed.). 1864–1866. *Leechdoms, Wortcunning and Starcraft of Early England (containing Peri didaxeon)*. 3 vols. (*Rolls Series* 35). London: Rerum Britannicarum Medii Ævi Scriptores.

Fleischhacker, Robert von (ed.). 1894. *Lanfrank's "Science of Cirurgie"*. (*EETS, OS* 102). London: Kegan Paul, Trench, Trübner and Co.

Getz, Faye M. 1991. *Healing and Society in Medieval England. A Middle English Translation of the Pharmaceutical Writings of Gilbertus Anglicus*. Wisconsin: Wisconsin University Press.

Hallaert, M.R. (ed.). 1982. *The "Sekenesse of wymmen". A Middle English Treatise on Diseases in Women*. (*Scripta: Mediaeval and Renaissance Texts and Studies* 8). Brussels: Omirel.

Power, d'Arcy (ed.). 1910. *John Arderne: Treatises of Fistula in Ano. Haemorrhoids and Clysters*. (*EETS, OS* 139). London: Oxford University Press.

Rowland, Beryl. 1981. *Medieval Woman's Guide to Health. The First English Gynaecological Handbook*. Kent: Kent State University Press.

Taavitsainen, Irma — Päivi Pahta — Martti Mäkinen (eds.). 2005. *Middle English Medical Texts* (*MEMT*). CD-ROM. Amsterdam: John Benjamins.

de Vriend, Hubert Jan (ed.). 1984. *The Old English Herbarium and Medicina de Quadrupedibus*. (*EETS OS* 286). London: Oxford University Press.

Wallner, Björn (ed.). 1964a. *The Middle English Translation of Guy de Chauliac's "Anatomy", with Guy's Essay on the History of Medicine*. (Lunds Universitets Årsskrift, N. F. 1, Vol. 56, No. 5.). Lund: Gleerup.

Wallner, Björn (ed.). 1969. *The Middle English Translation of Guy de Chauliac's Treatise on Fractures and Dislocations: Book 5 of the Great Surgery*. Lund: Gleerup.

Wallner, Björn (ed.). 1971. *A Middle English Version of the Introduction to Guy de Chauliac's "Chirurgia Magna"*. (*Acta Universitatis Lundensis, Sectio I. Theologica, juridica, humaniora*, 12). Lund: Gleerup.

Wallner, Björn (ed.). 1976. *The Middle English Translation of Guy de Chauliac's "Treatise on Wounds: Book III of the Great Surgery"*. (*Acta Universitatis Lundensis, Sectio I. Theologica, juridica, humaniora*, 23). Lund: Gleerup.

Wallner, Björn (ed.). 1982. *The Middle English Translation of Guy de Chauliac's Treatise on Ulcers*. Stockholm: Almqvist and Wiksell.

(c) Special studies

Ackerknecht, Erwin H. 2016. *A Short History of Medicine*. Baltimore: Johns Hopkins University Press.

Adams, Valerie. 1982. *An Introduction to Modern English Word-Formation*. Harlow: Longman.

Algeo, John — Carmen A. Butcher. 2013. *The Origins and Development of the English Language*. Boston: Wadsworth.

Allen, Loyd V. — Howard C. Ansel. 2013. *Ansel's Pharmaceutical Dosage Forms and Drug Delivery Systems*. 10th edition. Philadelphia/Baltimore/New York/London: Wolters Kluwer/Lippincott Williams & Wilkins.

Alonso Almeida, Francisco. 1998. "*As it ys seyde to fore*. Some linguistic evidence in the process of compiling Middle English recipes". *Selim. Journal of the Spanish Society for Mediaeval English Language and Literature* 8: 171–191.

Alonso Almeida, Francisco. 1999. "*Gyf hyr this medycyn*. Analysing the Middle English medical recipe discourse". *Revista de Lenguas para Fines Específicos* 5–6: 49–81.

Alonso Almeida, Francisco. 2008. "The Middle English medical charm: Register, genre and text type variables". *Neuphilologische Mitteilungen* 109.1: 9–38.

Alonso Almeida, Francisco. 2013. "Genre conventions in English recipes (1600–1800)". In: Michelle DiMeo — Sara Pennell (eds.) *Reading and Writing Recipe Books 1550–1800*. Manchester: Manchester University Press. 68–92.

Alonso Almeida, Francisco — Mercedes Cabrera-Cabreu. 2002. "The formulation of promise in medieval English medical recipes: A relevance-theoretic approach". *Neophilologus* 96: 137–154.

Alonso Almeida, Francisco — Ruth Carroll. 2004. "A new proposal for the classification of Middle English medical texts". In: Alicia Rodríguez-Álvarez — Francisco Alonso Almeida (eds.) *Voices on the Past: Studies in Old and Middle English Language and Literature*. A Coruña: Netbiblo. 21–33.

Alves, Rômulo R. N. — Ierecê L. Rosa (eds.). 2013. *Animals in Traditional Folk Medicine*. Berlin/Heidelberg: Springer-Verlag.

Amundsen, Darrel W. 1996. *Medicine, Society, and Faith in the Ancient and Medieval Worlds*. Baltimore: The John Hopkins University Press.

Anderson, Stuart. 2005. *Making Medicines. A Brief History of Pharmacy and Pharmaceuticals*. London/Chicago: Pharmaceutical Press.

Annual Bibliography of English Language and Literature (ABELL): online edition, available at http://www.proquest.com/products-services/abell.html (date of access: June – September 2017).

Bakhtiar, Laleh — Samira Ardalan. 2014. *Mysteries of the Apostles' Ointment from the Formula in Avicenna'a Canon of Medicine*. Chicago: Kazi Publications Incorporated.

Bately, Janet. 1996. "Towards a Middle English thesaurus: Some terms relating to FORTUNE, FATE and CHANCE". In: Jacek Fisiak (ed.) *Middle English Miscellany: From Vocabulary to Linguistic Variation*. Poznań: Motivex. 69–82.

Bately, Janet. 2000. "*Here comes the judge:* A small contribution to the study of French input into the vocabulary of the law in Middle English". In: Irma Taavitsainen — Terttu Nevelainen — Päivi Pahta — Matti Rissanen (eds.) *Placing Middle English in Context*. Berlin/New York: Mouton de Gruyter. 255–275.

Bator, Magdalena. 2006. "Scandinavian loanwords in English in the 15th century". *Studia Anglica Posnaniensia* 42: 285–299.

Bator, Magdalena. 2009a. "Obsolete Scandinavian loanwords in English – a semantic analysis of the field 'people'". *Kwartalnik Neofilologiczny* 56.3: 339–347.

Bator, Magdalena. 2009b. "Sense and inventory changes in the semantic field 'smell' in the history of English". *Inozemna Philologia* 121: 72–79.

Bator, Magdalena. 2010. *Obsolete Scandinavian Loanwords in English* (*Studies in English Medieval Language and Literature* 26). Frankfurt am Main: Peter Lang.

Bator, Magdalena. 2011. "French culinary vocabulary in the 14th-century English". In: Jacek Fisiak — Magdalena Bator (eds.) *Foreign Influences on Medieval English* (*Studies in English Medieval Language and Literature* 28). Frankfurt am Main: Peter Lang Verlag. 287–301.

Bator, Magdalena. 2012. "The semantic field TASTE in Old and Middle English". *Medieval English Mirror* 8: 89–102.

Bator, Magdalena. 2013a. "Verbs of cooking in Middle English: *Fry*, *roast* and *bake*". In: Jacek Fisiak — Magdalena Bator (eds.) *Historical English Word-formation and Semantics* (*Warsaw Studies in English Language and Literature* 15.). Frankfurt am Main: Peter Lang Verlag. 125–138.

Bator, Magdalena. 2013b. "Boil vs. seethe in Middle English". In: Liliana Sikorska — Marcin Krygier (eds.) *Evur happie & glorious, ffor I hafe at will grete riches* (*Medieval English Mirror* 9). Frankfurt am Main: Peter Lang Verlag. 27–40.

Bator, Magdalena. 2013c. "Sugar and spice and all things nice – an analysis of the culinary vocabulary in Middle English". *Kwartalnik Neofilologiczny* 60.4: 425–439.

Bator, Magdalena. 2014. *Culinary Verbs in Middle English*. Frankfurt am Main: Peter Lang Verlag.

Bator, Magdalena. 2015. "Foreign influences on the language of cookery in Middle English". *Kwartalnik Neofilologiczny* 62.4: 567–584.

Bator, Magdalena — Marta Sylwanowicz. 2016. "Recipe, receipt and prescription in the history of English". *Selim. Journal of the Spanish Society for Medieval English Language and Literature* 21: 1–23.

Bator, Magdalena — Marta Sylwanowicz. 2017a. "Measures in medieval English recipes - culinary vs. medical". *Studia Anglica Posnaniensia* 52.1: 21–52.

Bator, Magdalena — Marta Sylwanowicz. 2017b. "The typology of medieval recipes - culinary vs. medical". In: Jacek Fisiak — Magdalena Bator — Marta Sylwanowicz (eds.) *Essays and Studies in Middle English*. Frankfurt am Main: Peter Lang Verlag. 11–33.

Bator, Magdalena — Marta Sylwanowicz. 2017c. "Once you see it, once you don't - the case of null objects in Middle English culinary and medical recipes". In: Artur Kijak — Andrzej M. Łęcki — Jerzy Nykiel (eds.) *Current Developments in English Historical Linguistics. Studies in Honour of Rafał Molencki*. Katowice: Wydawnictwo Universytetu Śląskiego. 51–67.

Bauer, Laurie. 2002. *English Word-Formation*. Cambridge: Cambridge University Press.

Baugh, Albert C. 1935. "The chronology of loan-words in English". *Modern Language Notes* 50: 90–93.

Baugh, Albert C. — Thomas Cable. 1978. *A History of the English Language*. 3rd edition. Englewood Cliffs: Prentice-Hall, Inc.

Beck, Theodore R. 1974. *The Cutting Edge. Early History of the Surgeons of London*. London: Lund Humphries.

Benson, Larry (ed.). 2000. *The Canterbury Tales, Complete/Geoffrey Chaucer*. Boston: Houghton Mifflin.

Biber, Douglas. 1988. *Variation Across Speech and Writing*. Cambridge: Cambridge University Press.

Biber, Douglas — Victoria Clark. 2002. "Historical shifts in modification patterns with complex noun phrase structures". In: Teresa Fanego — Javier Pérez-Guerra — José López-Couso (eds.) *English Historical Syntax and Morphology*. Amsterdam: Benjamins. 43–66.

Blake, Norman (ed.). 1992. *The Cambridge History of the English Language*. Vol. 2.: 1066–1476. Cambridge: Cambridge University Press.

Bullough, Vern L. 1961. "Medical study at mediaeval Oxford". *Speculum* 36: 600–612.

Bullough, Vern L. 1962. "The medieval medical school at Cambridge". *Medieval Studies* 24: 161–168.

Bullough, Vern L. 1966. *The Development of Medicine As a Profession.* Basel: S. Karger.

Cameron, Malcolm L. 1993. *Anglo-Saxon Medicine.* Cambridge: Cambridge University Press.

Cameron, Angus — Allison Kingsmill — Ashley C. Amos. 1983. *Old English Word Studies: A Preliminary Author and Word Index.* Toronto: University of Toronto Press.

Carroll, Ruth. 1997. Cooking Verbs in Fourteenth-century English: A Semantic Class and Its Syntactic Behaviour. Unpublished Ph.D. dissertation: University of Oxford.

Carroll, Ruth. 1999. "The Middle English recipe as a text type". *Neuphilologische Mitteilungen* 100: 27–42.

Carroll, Ruth. 2004. "Middle English recipes: Vernacularisation of a text-type". In: Irma Taavitsainen — Päivi Pahta (eds.) *Medical and Scientific Writing in Late Medieval English* (*Studies in English Language*). Cambridge: Cambridge University Press. 174–191.

Carrillo-Linares, Maria J. 2005. "Middle English *Antidotarium Nicholai*: Evidence for linguistic distribution and dissemination in the vernacular". *International Journal of English Studies* 5.2: 75–96.

Cartwright, Frederick F. 1986. *A Social History of Medicine.* London/New York: Longman.

Carver, Craig M. 1991. *A History of English in Its Own Words.* New York: Harper Collins Publishers.

Chambers, Mark C. 2009. "'What is this, a betel, or a batowe, or a buskin lacyd?' Lexicological confusion in medieval clothing culture". In: Javier E. Díaz Vera — Rosario Caballero Rodríguez (eds.) *Textual Healing: Studies in Medieval English Medical, Scientific and Technical Texts.* (*Linguistic Insights: Studies in Language and Communication* 101). Bern: Peter Lang. 55–74.

Chambers, Mark C. 2017. "How long is a *launce*? Units of measure for cloth in late medieval and Early Modern Britain". In: Robin Netherton — Gale Owen-Crocker (eds.) *Medieval Clothing and Textiles.* Vol. 13. Woodbridge: Boydell and Brewer. 31–66.

Chambers, Mark C. — Gale Owen-Crocker. (2008). "From head to hand to arm: The lexicological history of 'cuff'". In: Robin Netherton — Gale Owen-Crocker (eds.) *Medieval Clothing and Textiles.* Vol. 4. Woodbridge: Boydell and Brewer. 55–67.

Chambers, Mark C. — Louise M. Sylvester. 2010a. "Multilingualism in the vocabulary of dress and textiles in late medieval Britain". In: Iren Hegerdüs — Alexandra Fodor (eds.) *English Historical Linguistics 2010.* (*Current Issues in*

Linguistic Theory 325). Amsterdam/Philadelphia: John Benjamins Publishing Company. 313–326.

Chambers, Mark C. — Louise M. Sylvester. 2010b. "Lexicological confusion and medieval clothing culture: redressing medieval dress with the Lexis of Cloth and Clothing in Britain Project". In: Tara Hamling — Catherine Richardson (eds.) *Everyday Objects: Medieval and Early Modern Material Culture and Its Meanings*. Burlington/Aldershot: Ashgate. 71–78.

Chambers, Mark C. — Louise M. Sylvester. 2010c. "From apareil to warderobe: some observations on Anglo-French in the Middle English". In: Richard Ingham (ed.) *The Anglo-Norman Language and Its Contexts*. York: York Medieval Press. 63–73.

Charen, Thelma. 1951. "The etymology of medicine". *Bulletin of the Medical Library Association* 39.3: 216–221.

Chaudhary, Umair J. — John S. Duncan — Louis Lemieux. 2011. "A dialogue with historical concepts of epilepsy from the Babylonians to Hughlings Jackson: Persisten beliefs". *Epilepsy and Behavior* 21.2: 109–114.

Cholmeley, Henry P. 1912. *John of Gaddesden and the Rosa Medicinae*. Oxford: Clarendon Press.

Ciszek, Ewa. 2013. "Middle English decline of the Old English lēode: A case study of the manuscripts of Laȝamon's Brut". In: Jacek Fisiak — Magdalena Bator (eds.) *Historical English Word-Formation and Semantics* (*Warsaw Studies in Engish Language and Literature* 15). Frankfurt am Main: Peter Lang Verlag. 229–243.

Coleman, Julie. 1996. "The treatment of sexual vocabulary in Middle English dictionaries". In: Jacek Fisiak (ed.) *Middle English Miscellany: From Vocabulary to Linguistic Variation*. Poznań: Motivex. 183–206.

Conrad, Lawrence I. — Michael Neve et al. 2011. *The Western Medical Tradition: 800 BC to AD 1800*. Cambridge: Cambridge University Press.

Crespo García, Begoña — Isabel Moskowich-Spiegel. 2004. "Enlarging the lexicon: The field of technology and administration from 1150 to 1500". *Studia Anglica Posnaniensia* 40: 163–181.

Cruz-Cabanillas, Isabel. 2017. "Medical recipes in Glasgow University Library Manuscript Fergusson 147". In: Jacek Fisiak — Magdalena Bator — Marta Sylwanowicz (eds.) *Essays and Studies in Middle English*. Frankfurt am Main: Peter Lang Verlag. 77–94.

Crystal, David. 2006. *The Cambridge Encyclopedia of the English Language*. Cambridge: Cambridge University Press.

Cummings, Michael. 1980. "Paired opposites in Wulfstan's Sermo Lupi ad Anglos". *Revue de l'Université d'Ottawa* 50: 233–243.

Dalton-Puffer, Christiane. 1996. *The French Influence on Middle English Morphology. A Corpus-Based Study of Derivation.* Berlin/New York: Mouton de Gruyter.

Daly, Walter J. — Robert D. Yee. 2001. "The eye book of Master Peter of Spain: A glimpse of diagnosis and treatment of eye disease in the Middle Ages". *Documenta Ophtalmologica* 103: 119–153.

Dance, Richard. 2003. *Words derived from Old Norse in Early Middle English: Studies in the vocabulary of the South-West Midland texts.* (*Medieval and Renaissance Texts and Studies* 246). Tempe: Arizona Center for Medieval and Renaissance Studies.

Dash, Alekha — Somnath Singh — Justin Tolman (eds.). 2013. *Pharmaceutics: Basic Principles and Application to Pharmacy Practice.* San Diego/London/Waltham: Academic Press.

Dekeyser, Xavier. 1991. "Romance loans in in Late Middle English: a case study". In: Sylviane Granger (ed.) *Perspectives on the English Lexicon: A Tribute to Jacques van Roey* (*Cahiers de l'Institut de Linguistique de Louvain* 17). Louvain-la-Neuve: Cabay. 153–162.

Dekeyser, Xavier. 1995. "*Travel*, *journey* and *voyage* – an exploration into the realm of Middle English lexico-semantics". *NOWELE: North-Western European Language Evolution* 25: 127–136.

Dickson, Keith. 1998. *Stephanus the Philosopher and Physician. Commentary on Galen's Therapeutics to Glaucon.* Leiden/Boston/Köln: Brill.

Diensberg, Bernhard. 1985. "The lexical fields boy/girl – servant – child in Middle English". *Neuphilologische Mitteilungen* 3: 328–336.

Diller, Hans-Jürgen. 1996. "*Joy* and *mirth* in Middle English (and a little bit in Old): A plea for the consideration of genre in historical semantics". In: Jacek Fisiak (ed.) *Middle English Miscellany: From Vocabulary to Linguistic Variation.* Poznań: Motivex. 83–105.

Diller, Hans-Jürgen. 2011. "Why ANGER and JOY? Were TĒNE and BLISS not good enough?". In: Jacek Fisiak — Magdalena Bator (eds.) *Foreign Influences on Medieval English.* Frankfurt am Main: Peter Lang Verlag. 213–230.

Dirckx, John H. 1983. *The Language of Medicine. Its Evolution, Structure, and Dynamics.* 2nd edition. New York: Praeger.

Dobrovolska, Oksana. 2017. "The names of herdsmen in the Middle English language: Historical development of the lexical-thematic group". *Studies About Languages* 30: 73–89.

Durkin, Philip. 2014. *Borrowed Words. A History of Loanwords in English.* Oxford: Oxford University Press.

van Dyke, Carolynn. 2012. "Names of the beasts: Tracking the *animot* in medieval texts". *Studies in the Age of Chaucer* 34: 1–51.

Edelstein, Emma J. — Ludwig Edelstein. 1998. *Asclepius: Collection and Interpretation of the Testimonies*. Baltimore: Johns Hopkins University Press.

Eldredge, Laurence M. 1996. *Benvenutus Grassus; The Wonderful Art of the Eye: A Critical Edition of the Middle English Translation of his De probatissima arte oculorum*. East Lansing: Michigan State University.

Eldredge, Laurence M. 1998. "A thirteenth-century ophthalmologist, Benvenutus Grassus: His treatise and its survival". *Journal of the Royal Society of Medicine* 91: 47–52.

Eldredge, Laurence M. 1999. "The English vernacular afterlife of Benvenutus Grassus, ophthalmologist". *Early Science and Medicine* 4.2: 149–163.

Enciclopedia Italiana di Scienze, Lettere ed Arti (Italian Encyclopaedia of Science, Letters, and Arts). 1929–2015. Online edition available at http://www.treccani.it (date of access: August 2017).

Esquibel, Joanna. 2015. "How would they *transfer* the message across? From *wendan* to *translaten*: On the replacement of native forms with Romance borrowing". *Anglica* 24.2: 79–102.

Esquibel, Joanna — Anna Wojtyś. 2012. "Devil *aka* Satan: an *enemy* or *fiend*? On the rivalry between the familiar and the foreign in early English". *Token: A Journal of English Linguistics* 1: 97–113.

Esteve Ramos, Maria J. 2008. *English Medical Vocabulary in Ophthalmology: A Historical Review*. München: Lincom Europa.

Fabiszak, Małgorzata. 2001. *The Concept of 'Joy' in Old and Middle English. A Semantic Analysis*. Piła: Wyższa Szkoła Biznesu.

Fennel, Barbara. 2001. *A History of English: A Sociolinguistic Approach*. (*Blackwell Textbooks in Linguistics*, 1st edition). Oxford: Blackwell.

Filipowicz, Natalia. 2010. "Tracing the origins and fates of African fauna vocabulary in Middle English". In: Jacek Fisiak (ed.) *Studies in Old and Middle English* (*Warsaw Studies in English Language and Literature* 1). Łódź/Warszawa: SWSPiZ. 91–105.

Fischer, Olga. 2004. "Developments in the category adjective from Old to Middle English". *Studies in Medieval Language and Literature* 19: 1–36.

Fischer, Olga. 2006. "On the position of adjectives in Middle English". *English Language and Linguistics* 10.2: 253–288.

Fisiak, Jacek. 1977. *Bibliography of Writings on English Language and Literature in Poland* (*1945–1975*). Warsaw: PWN.

Fisiak, Jacek. 1983. *A Bibliography of Writings for the History of the English Language.* Poznań: Wydawnictwo Naukowe UAM.

Fisiak, Jacek. 2000. *An Outline History of English. Volume One. External History.* 3rd edition. Poznań: Wydawnictwo Poznańskie.

Frantzen, Allen J. 2011. "Food words in the Anglo-Saxon penitentials". In: Renate Bauer — Ulrike Krischke (eds.) *More Than Words: English Lexicography and Lexicology Past and Present. Essays Presented to Hans Sauer on the Occasion of his 65th Birthday.* 2 parts. (*Münchener Universitätsschriften* 36). Frankfurt am Main: Peter Lang Verlag. 83–99.

French, Roger. 2003. *Medicine Before Science. The Business of Medicine from the Middle Ages to the Enlightenment.* Cambridge: Cambridge University Press.

Fries, Charles C. 1938. "Some notes on the inflected genitive in Present-day English". *Language* 14: 121–133.

Fries, Charles. C. 1940. "On the development of the structural use of word-order in Modern English". *Language* 16: 199–208.

Garcia, Antonio M. — Santiago G. Fernández-Corugedo. (eds.). 2011. *Benvenutus Grassus' On the Well-proven Art of the Eye: "Practica Oculorum & De probatissima Arte Oculorum".* (*Late Middle English Texts* 1). Berna: Peter Lang.

Garcia-Ballester, Luis — Roger French — Jon Arrizabalaga — Andrew Cunningham (eds.). 1994. *Practical Medicine from Salerno to the Black Death.* Cambridge/New York: Cambridge University Press.

Gasbarro, Ron. October 2005. "It was all Greek to them". The Bowl of Hygeia. A Supplement to Drug Topics, 1–2.

Gerald, Michael C. 2013. *The Drug Book. From Arsenic to Xanax, 250 Milestones in the History of Drugs.* New York: Sterling.

Gerard, John. 2015. [1633] *The Herbal or General History of Plants: The Complete 1633 Edition as Revised and Enlarged by Thomas Johnson.* New York: Calla Editions.

Getz, Faye M. 1990. "Medical practitioners in medieval England". *Social History of Medicine* 3: 245–283.

Getz, Faye M. 1998. *Medicine in the English Middle Ages.* Princeton: Princeton University Press.

Görlach, Manfred. 1992. "Text-types and language history: The cookery recipe". In: Matti Rissanen — Ossi Ihalainen — Terttu Nevalainen — Irma Taavitsainen (eds.) *History of Englishes: New Methods and Interpretations in Historical Linguistics.* Berlin/New York: Mouton de Gruyter. 736–761.

Görlach, Manfred. 1993. *Introduction to Early Modern English.* Cambridge: Cambridge University Press.

Green, James. 2000a. *The Herbal Medicine-Maker's Handbook. A Home Manual.* New York: Crossing Press.

Green, Monica H. 1989. "Women's medical practice and medical care in medieval Europe". *Signs* 14: 434–473.

Green, Monica H. 2000b. "Books as a source of medical education for women in the Middle Ages". *Dynamis: Acta Hispanica ad Medicinae Scientiarumque Historiam Illustrandam* 20: 331–69.

Green, Monica H. 2000c "From 'diseases of women' to 'secrets of women': The transformation of gynecological literature in the later Middle Ages". *Journal of Medieval and Early Modern Studies* 30: 5–39.

Green, Monica H. 2000d. *Women's Healthcare in the Medieval West: Texts and Contexts* (*Variorum Collected Studies Series*, CS680). Aldershot: Ashgate.

Green, Monica H. 2001. (ed. and trans.). *The 'Trotula': A Medieval Compendium of Women's Medicine.* Philadelphia: University of Pennsylvania Press.

Green, Monica H. 2008. *Making Women's Medicine Masculine. The Rise of Male Authority in Pre-Modern Gynaecology.* Oxford: Oxford University Press.

Greilsammer, Myriam. 1991. "The midwife, the priest, and the physician". *Journal of Medieval and Renaissance Studies* 21: 285–329.

Griggs, Barbara. 1982. *Green Pharmacy. A History of Herbal Medicine.* London: Jill Norman & Hobhouse.

Grigsby, Bryon. 1996. "The social position of the surgeon in London, 1350–1450". *Proceedings of the Illinois Medieval Association: Essays in Medieval Studies* 13: 71–78.

Grygiel, Marcin. 2008. *From Semantic Change to Conceptual Blending. Semantic Development of English Historical Near-Synonyms of MAN/MALE HUMAN BEING.* Rzeszów: Wydawnictwo Uniwersytetu Rzeszowskiego.

Gustafsson, Marita. 1975. *Binomial Expressions in Present-Day English: A Syntactic and Semantic Study.* Turku: Turun Yliopisto.

Haubrich, William S. 1997. *Medical Meanings. A Glossary of Word Origin.* Philadelphia: American College of Physicians.

Hogg, Richard — David Denison (eds.). 2008. *A History of the English Language.* Cambridge: Cambridge University Press.

Hughes, Geoffrey. 1988. *Words in Time: A Social History of the English Vocabulary.* Oxford: Blackwell.

Hughes, Geoffrey. 2000. *A History of English Words.* Oxford: Blackwell.

Hughes, Muriel J. 1943. *Women Healers in Medieval Life and Literature.* New York: King's Crown Press.

Hunt, Tony. 1989. *Plant Names in Medieval England.* Cambridge: D.S. Brewer.

Hunt, Tony. 1990. *Popular Medicine in Thirteenth-century England: Introduction and Texts*. Cambridge: D. S. Brewer.

Hunt, Tony. 1999. *The Medieval Surgery*. Woodbridge: The Boydell Press.

Jespersen, Otto. 1972 [1905]. *Growth and Structure of the English Language*. Leipzig: Trübner.

Jones, Claire. 1998a. "Formula and formulation: "Efficacy phrases" in medieval English medical manuscripts". *Neuphilologische Mitteilungen* 99: 199–209.

Jones, Peter M. 1984. *Medieval Medical Miniatures*. London: British Library.

Jones, Peter M. 1989. "Four Middle English translations of John Arderne". In: Alastair J. Minnis (ed.) *Latin and Vernacular: Studies in Late-Medieval Texts and Manuscripts*. Cambridge: D.S. Brewer. 61–89.

Jones, Peter M. 1994. "John of Arderne and the Mediterranean tradition of scholastic surgery". In: Luis García-Ballester — Roger French — Jon Arrizabalaga — Andrew Cunningham (eds.) *Practical Medicine from Salerno to the Black Death*. Cambridge/New York: Cambridge University Press. 289–321.

Jones, Peter M. 1998b. "Thomas Fayreford: An English fifteenth-century medical practitioner". In: Roger French — Jon Arrizabalaga — Andrew Cunningham — Luis García-Ballester (eds.) *Medicine from the Black Death to the French Disease*. (*History of Medicine in Context Series*). Aldershot: Ashgate. 156–183.

Karczmarczyk, Justyna. 2011. "In the realm of fantasy: *wyrm/worm* vs. *draca* and *dragon* in Medieval English". In: Jacek Fisiak — Magdalena Bator (eds.) *Foreign Influences on Medieval English*. Frankfurt am Main: Peter Lang Verlag. 155–165.

Karczmarczyk, Justyna. 2012. "Three terms denoting dragons in Middle English poetry and prose: *dragon, drake* and *worm*". In: Joanna Esquibel — Anna Wojtyś (eds.) *Explorations in the English Language: Middle Ages and Beyond. Festschrift for Professor Jerzy Wełna on the Occasion of his 70th Birthday*. Frankfurt am Main: Peter Lang. 257–265.

Kaunisto, Mark. 2009. "Rivalry between English adjectives in *-ive* and *-ory*". In: Rod McConchie — Alpo Honkapohja — Jukka Tyrkkö (eds.) *Selected Proceedings of the* 2008 *Symposium on New Approaches in English Historical Lexis*. Somerville: Cascadilla Press. 74–87.

Kennedy, Arthur G. 1927. *A Bibliography of Writings on the English Language from the Beginning of Printing to the End of 1922*. Harvard: Harvard University Press.

Kiełtyka, Robert. 2008. *On Zoosemy: The Study of Middle English and Early Modern English DOMESTICATED ANIMALS*. Rzeszów: Wydawnictwo Uniwersytetu Rzeszowskiego.

King James Bible: online edition available at https://www.kingjamesbibleonline.org (date of access: June – September 2017).

Kjellmer, Göran. 1973. *Middle English Words for 'People'*. (*Gothenburg Studies in English* 27). Stockholm: Almqvist & Wiksell.

Kleparski, Grzegorz. 1997. *Theory and Practice of Historical Semantics: The Case of Middle English and Early Modern English Synonyms of GIRL/YOUNG WOMAN*. Lublin: The University Press of the Catholic University of Lublin.

Kleparski, Grzegorz. 2005. "Towards the semantics of Middle English synonyms of MAN". *Studia Anglica Resoviensia* 3.25: 88–95.

Kłos, Małgorzata. 2010. "'To die' in early Middle English: *deien*, *swelten* or *sterven*?" In: Jacek Fisiak (ed.) *Studies in Old and Middle English* (*Warsaw Studies in English Language and Literature* 1). Łódź/Warszawa: SWSPiZ. 155–164.

Knowles, Gerry. 1997. *A Cultural History of the English Language*. London/New York: Arnold.

Kohl, Norbert. 1970. *Bibliographie für das Studium der Anglistik*. Bad Homburg: Athenäum Verlag.

Kopaczyk, Joanna. 2009. "(Multi-word) units of meaning in 16th-century legal Scots". In: Rod McConchie — Alpo Honkapohja — Jukka Tyrkkö (eds.) *Selected Proceedings of the* 2008 *Symposium on New Approaches in English Historical Lexis*. Somerville: Cascadilla Proceedings Project. 88–95.

Kopaczyk, Joanna. 2013. *The Legal Language of Scottish Burghs: Standardization and Lexical Bundles (1380–1560)*. Oxford: Oxford University Press.

Kopaczyk, Joanna — Hans Sauer. 2017. *Binomials in the History of English*. Cambridge: Cambridge University Press.

Kornexl, Lucia — Ursula Lenker. 2011. "Culinary and other pairs: Lexical borrowing and conceptual differentiation in Early English food terminology". In: Renate Bauer — Ulrike Krischke (eds.) *More Than Words: English Lexicography and Lexicology Past and Present. Essays Presented to Hans Sauer on the Occasion of his 65th Birthday*. 2 parts. (*Münchener Universitätsschriften* 36). Frankfurt am Main: Peter Lang Verlag. 179–206.

Koskenniemi, Inna. 1968. *Repetitive Word Pairs in Old and Middle English Prose. Expressions of the Type Whole and Sound and Answered and Said, and Other Parallel Constructions*. (*Annales Universitatis Turkuensis*, Ser. B, Tom. 107). Turku: University of Turku.

Koziol, Herbert. 1972. *Handbuch der englischen Wortbildungslehre*. 2nd edition. Heidelberg: Winter.

Kruse, Britta-Juliane. 1996. *Verborgene Heilkünste. Geschichte der Frauenmedizin im Spätmittelalter*. Berlin/New York: Walter de Gruyter.

Kruse, Britta-Juliane. 1999. *"Die Arznei ist Goldes wert". Mittelalterliche Frauenrezepte.* Berlin/New York: Walter de Gruyter.

Krygier, Marcin. 2012. "Vernacularisation of the lexicon in the Wycliffe Bible: The Book of Ruth in MSS. CCC 4 and BL Royal I. C. VIII". In: Joanna Esquibel — Anna Wojtyś (eds.) *Explorations in the English Language: Middle Ages and Beyond. Festschrift for Professor Jerzy Wełna on the Occasion of his 70th Birthday.* Frankfurt am Main: Peter Lang. 199–209.

Lang, Sheila J. 1998. The "Philomena" of John Bradmore and its Middle English derivative: A perspective on surgery in Late Medieval England. Doctoral dissertation. University of St. Andrews.

Leisi, Ernst. 1947. *Die tautologischen Wortpaare in Caxton's Eneydos: Zur synchronischen Bedeutungs- und Ursachenforschung.* Cambridge: Murray.

Leisi, Ernst — Christian Mair. 1999. *Das heutige Englisch: Wesenszüge und Probleme.* 8th edition. Heidelberg: Winter.

Lindberg, David C. — Michael H. Shank (eds.). 2015. *The Cambridge History of Science: Volume 2, Medieval Science.* Cambridge: Cambridge University Press.

Lipka, Leonhard. 1992. *An Outline of English Lexicology. Lexical Structure, Word Semantics, and Word-Formation.* Tübingen: Max Niemeyer Verlag.

Łodej, Sylwester. 2012. "Semantic change in the domain of the vocabulary of Christian clergy". In: Hans Sauer — Gaby Waxenberger (eds.) *English Historical Linguistics* (*Current Issues in Linguistic Theory* 324). Amsterdam: John Benjamins. 99–115.

MacKinney, Loren C. 1946. "Animal substances in materia medica". *Journal of the History of Medicine and Allied Sciences* 1.1: 149–170.

Malkiel, Yakov. 1959. "Studies in irreversible binomials". *Lingua* 8: 113–160.

Marchand, Hans. 1969. *The Categories and Types of Present-Day English Word-Formation.* 2nd edition. München: Verlag C.H. Beck.

Markus, Manfred. 2008. "The topos of *foul/filth* in Middle English homilies: A study in historical lexicology". *Neuphilologische Mitteilungen* 109: 223–240.

Marriott, John F. — Keith A. Wilson — Christopher A. Langley — Dawn Belcher. 2010. *Pharmaceutical Compounding and Dispensing.* 2nd edition. London: Pharmaceutical Press.

Matheson, Lister M. (ed.). 1994. *Popular and Practical Science of Medieval England.* East Lansing: Colleagues Press.

Matthews, Leslie G. 1962. *History of Pharmacy in Britain.* Edinburgh/London: E. & S. Livingstone Ltd.

Mayer, Johannes G. 2008. *Das geheime Heilwissen der Klosterfrauen.* Reinbek bei Hamburg: Rowohlt Verlag GmbH.

Mayer, Johannes G. 2010. *Tajemnice Sztuki Medycznej Średniowiecznych Zakonnic*. Kraków: Wydawnictwo WAM.

Mäkinen, Matti. 2004. "Herbal recipes and recipes in herbals: Intertextuality in Early English medical writing". In: Irma Taavitsainen — Päivi Pahta (eds.) *Medical and Scientific Writing in Late Medieval English*. Cambridge: Cambridge University Press. 144–173.

Mäkinen, Matti. 2006. Between Herbals et Alia: Intertextuality in Medieval English Herbals. PhD dissertation, University of Helsinki, Faculty of Arts, Department of English and the Research Unit for Variation, Contacts and Change in English.

McConchie, Roderick W. 1997. *Lexicography and Physicke: The Record of Sixteenth-Century English Medical Terminology*. Oxford: Clarendon Press.

Meroney, Howard. 1945. "Irish in the Old English charms". *Speculum* 20: 172–182.

Miller, Gary D. 2006. *Latin Suffixal Derivatives in English and their Indo-European Ancestry*. Oxford: Oxford University Press.

Miller, Gary D. 2012. *External Influences on English: From Its Beginnings to the Renaissance*. Oxford: Oxford University Press.

Mills, Anthony D. 1968. "Notes on some Middle English occupational terms". *Studia Neophilologica* 40: 35–48.

Millward, Celia M. 1996. *A Biography of the English Language*. 2nd edition. Boston: Thomson Wadsworth.

Minkova, Donka — Robert Stockwell. 2009. *English Words: History and Structure*. Cambridge: Cambridge University Press.

Minnis, Alastair J. 1987. *The Medical Boethius: Studies in the Vernacular Translations of* De Consolatione Philosophiae. Cambridge: D.S. Brewer.

Miura, Ayumi. 2015. *Middle English Verbs of Emotion and Impersonal Constructions: Verb Meaning and Syntax in Diachrony*. Oxford: Oxford University Press.

Molencki, Rafał. 2015. "The competition between *purveyen* and *providen* in Late Middle English". In: Juan Camilo Conde-Silvestre — Javier Calle-Martín (eds.) *Approaches to Middle English. Variation, Contact and Change*. Frankfurt am Main/New York: Peter Lang. 67–82.

Molencki, Rafał. 2018. "Why did people oust *folk* and *lede*?". In: Michiko Ogura — Hans Sauer (eds.) *Medieval English Language and Literature*. Frankfurt: Peter Lang. 263–277.

Mollin, Sandra. 2014. *The (Ir)reversibility of English Binomials: Corpus, Constraints, Developments*. Amsterdam: John Benjamins.

Moskowich, Isabel. 2002. "The adjective in English. The 'French type' and its place in the history of the language". *Folia Linguistica Historica* 23.1–2: 59–71.

Moskowich, Isabel. 2009. "*Of medicineȝ sedatyueȝ*. Some notes on adjective position and oral register in Middle English medical texts". *Studia Anglica Posnaniensia* 45.1: 57–68.

Moskowich, Isabel — Begoña Crespo-Garcia. 2002. "Adjectival forms in Late Middle English. Syntactic and semantic implications". *Studia Neophilologica* 74: 161–170.

Müller-Schwefe, Gerhard. 1962. *Einführung in das Studium der englischen Philologie mit Bibliographie.* Tübingen: Niemeyer.

Newman, John G. 2006. "The borrowing of Latin and French nouns denoting Christian identities and its impact on Medieval English lexis and Medieval English religious writings". *Linguistica Bidgostiana* 3: 162–169.

Nockels-Fabbri, Christiane. 2007. "Treating medieval plague: The wonderful virtues of theriac". *Early Science and Medicine* 12: 247–283.

Norri, Juhani. 1987. Studies in the medical vocabulary of the fifteenth-century English. With special reference to four collections of medicinal recipes compiled around the middle of century. Unpublished licentiate thesis, University of Turku.

Norri, Juhani. 1989. "Premodification and postmodification as a means of term-formation in Middle English medical prose". *Neuphilologische Mitteilungen* 90: 147–162.

Norri, Juhani. 1992. *Names of Sicknesses in English,* 1400–1500*: An Exploration of the Lexical Field.* Helsinki: Suomalainen Tiedeakatemia.

Norri, Juhani. 1996. "On the origins of plant names in fifteenth-century English". In: Jacek Fisiak (ed.) *Middle English Miscellany: From Vocabulary to Linguistic Variation*. Poznań: Motivex. 159–181.

Norri, Juhani. 1998. *Names of Body Parts, 1400–1550.* Helsinki: Academia Scientiarum Fennicae.

Norri, Juhani. 2004. "Entrances and exits in English medical vocabulary, 1400–1550". In: Irma Taavitsainen — Päivi Pahta (eds.) *Medical and Scientific Writing in Late Medieval English.* Cambridge: Cambridge University Press. 100–143.

Nutton, Vivian. 2011. "Medicine in medieval western Europe, 1000–1500". In: Lawrence I. Conrad et al. (eds.) *The Western Medical Tradition, 800 BC to AD* 1800. Cambridge: Cambridge University Press.

O'Boyle, Cornelius. 1998. "The art of medicine: Medical teaching at the University of Paris, 1250–1400". In: Jürgen Miethke — William J. Courtenay —

Jeremy Catto — Jacque Verger (eds.) *Education and Society in the Middle Ages and Renaissance*. Vol. 9. Leiden/Boston/Köln: Brill.

Ogden, Margaret S. (ed.). 1971. *The Cyrurgie of Guy de Chauliac* (*Early English Text Society*, O.S. 265). London/New York/Toronto: Oxford University Press.

Ogura, Michiko. 1981. *The Syntactic and Semantic Rivalry of 'quoth', 'say', and 'tell' in Medieval English*. Hirakata City: Kufs Publication.

Ogura, Michiko. 2005. "*Afeard or afraid*? Rivalry and supersession". In: Jacek Fisiak - Hye-Kyung Kang (eds.) *Recent Trends in Medieval English Language and Literature in Honour of Young-Bae Park*. Vol. 1. Seoul: Thaehaksa Publishing Company. 189–201.

Ogura, Michiko. 2013. *Words and Expressions of Emotion in Medieval English* (*Studies in English Medieval Language and Literature* 39). Frankfurt am Main: Peter Lang.

Oizumi, Akio. 1966. *A Classified Bibliography of Writings on English Philology and Medieval English Literature*. Tokyo: Nan'un-Do.

Olszewska, Elizabeth S. 1935. "Legal borrowings from Norse in Old English and Middle English". *Saga - Book of the Viking Society* 11: 233–238.

Pahta, Päivi. 1998. *Medieval Embryology in the Vernacular: The Case of* De spermate (*Mémoires de la Société Néophilologique de Helsinki* 53). Helsinki: Société Néophilologique.

Pahta, Päivi. 2004. "Code-switching in medieval medical writing". In: Irma Taavitsainen — Päivi Pahta (eds.) *Medical and Scientific Writing in Late Medieval English*. Cambridge: Cambridge University Press. 73–99.

Pahta, Päivi — Irma Taavitsainen. 1995. "Authorities in medieval medical treatises". In: J.J. Mary Hatakka — Kirsti Peitsara (eds.) *The New Courant 3*. Helsinki: Department of English, University of Helsinki. 97–107.

Pahta, Päivi — Irma Taavitsainen. 2004. "Vernacularisation of scientific and medical writing in its sociohistorical context". In: Irma Taavitsainen — Päivi Pahta (eds.) *Medical and Scientific Writing in Late Medieval English*. Cambridge: Cambridge University Press. 1–22.

Palmer, James M. 2006. "Your malady is no "sodyn hap": Ophthalmology, Benvenutus Grassus, and January's blindness in the Merchant's Tale". *The Chaucer Review* 41.2: 197–205.

Pocuca, Marta — Dragan Stupar. 2006. "Pharmaceutical forms in *Antidotarium Nicolai*". *Macedonian Pharmaceutical Bulletin* 52.1–2: 49–56.

Porter, Roy. 2001. *The Cambridge Illustrated History of Medicine*. Cambridge: Cambridge University Press.

Pouchelle, Marie-Christine. 1990. *The Body and Surgery in the Middle Ages*. Cambridge: Rutgers University Press.

Power, Eileen. 1922. "Some women practitioners of medicine in the Middle Ages". *Proceedings of the Royal Society of Medicine* 15.6: 20–23.

Prins, Anton A. 1941–1942. "On the loss and substitution of words in Middle English". *Neophilologus* 26: 280–298, 27: 49–59.

Prioreschi, Plinio. 2003. *A History of Medicine*. Omaha: Horatius Press.

Pyles, Thomas — John Algeo. 2004. *The Origins and Development of the English Language*. 5th edition. Boston: Heinle & Heinle.

Quintana-Toledo, Elena. 2009. "Middle English medical recipes: A metadiscursive approach". *Studia Anglica Posnaniensia* 45.2: 21–38.

Raumolin-Brunberg, Helena. 1991. *The Noun Phrase in Early Sixteenth-century English: A Study Based on Sir Thomas More's Writings*. Helsinki: Societé Neophilologique.

Raumolin-Brunberg, Helena. 1994. "The position of adjectival modifiers in Late Middle English noun phrases". In: Udo Fries — Gunnel Tottie — Peter Schneider (eds.) *Creating and Using English Language Corpora*. Amsterdam: John Benjamins Publishing. 159–168.

Rawcliffe, Carole. 1995. *Medicine and Society in Later Medieval England*. Phoenix Mill: Alan Sutton.

Robbins, Rosel H. 1970. "Medical manuscripts in Middle English". *Speculum* 45: 393–415.

Roberts, Jane. 2000. "*Robbares and reuares þat ryche men despoilen*: Some competing forms". In: Irma Taavitsainen — Terttu Nevalainen — Päivi Pahta — Matti Rissanen (eds.) *Placing Middle English in Context*. Berlin/New York: Mouton de Gruyter. 229–253.

Rothwell, William. 1980. "Lexical borrowing in a Medieval context". *Bulletin of the John Rylands Library* 63.1: 118–143.

Rothwell, William. 1998. "Arrivals and departures: the adoption of French terminology into Middle English". *English Studies* 79: 155–165.

Rubin, Stanley. 1974. *Medieval English Medicine*. New York: Harper & Row.

Rusinek, Marietta. 2013. "Medieval French borrowings in English 'cakes' vocabulary: A historical semantic analysis". In: Liliana Sikorska — Marcin Krygier (eds.) *Evur happie & glorious, ffor I hafe at will grete riches* (*Medieval English Mirror* 9). Frankfurt am Main: Peter Lang Verlag. 61–70.

Rynell, Alarik. 1948. *The Rivalry of Scandinavian and Native Synonyms in Middle English Especially 'taken' and 'nimen', with an Excursus on Nema and Taka in Old Scandinavian*. (*Lund Studies in English* 13). Lund: Håkon Ohlssons Boktryckeri.

Sandahl, Bertil. 1951. *Middle English Sea Terms, Volume I: The Ship's Hull.* Upsala: Lundequistska Bokhandeln.

Sandahl, Bertil. 1959. *Middle English Sea Terms, Volume II: Masts, Spars and Sails*. Upsala: Lundequistska Bokhandeln.

Sandahl, Bertil. 1982. *Middle English Sea Terms, Volume III: Standing and Running Rigging.* (*Studia Anglistica Upsaliensia* 42). Upsala: Acta Universitatis Upsalensis.

Sauer, Hans. 1992. *Nominalkomposita im Frühmittelenglischen.* Tübingen: Max Niemeyer Verlag.

Sauer, Hans. 1996. "English plant names in the thirteenth century: The trilingual Harley vocabulary". In: Jacek Fisiak (ed.) *Middle English Miscellany: From Vocabulary to Linguistic Variation.* Poznań: Motivex. 135–155.

Sauer, Hans. 2011. "Patterns of loan-influence on the Medieval English plant names, with special reference to the influence of Greek". In: Jacek Fisiak — Magdalena Bator (eds.) *Foreign Influences on Medieval English.* Frankfurt am Main: Peter Lang Verlag. 55–76.

Sauer, Hans — David Scott-Macnab. 2017. "A thousand Middle English names for hunting hounds: Neologising, borrowing, and compounding in a 15th century list". In: Jacek Fisiak — Magdalena Bator — Marta Sylwanowicz (eds.) *Essays and Studies in Middle English.* Frankfurt am Main: Peter Lang Verlag. 163–197.

Savage, Henry L. 1951. "Hunting terms in Middle English". *Modern Language Notes* 66: 216.

Sayers, William. 1998. "The etymology of Middle English *oreven* 'oar blank.'". *Mariner's Mirror* 84.3: 322–325.

Sądej, Kinga. 2007. "The rivalry of native words and their French synonyms in Middle English: OE *beorg* and F *mountaine*". In: Piotr Stelmaszczyk — Iwona Witczak-Plisiecka (eds.) *PASE Studies in Linguistics.* Łódź: Wydawnictwo Uniwersytetu Łódzkiego. 263–275.

Sądej-Sobolewska, Kinga. 2011a. *The Synonyms of* Hill *and* Mountain *in Medieval English: Explorations in Historical Semantics.* (*Warsaw Studies in English Historical Linguistics* 5). Warsaw: Institute of English Studies, University of Warsaw.

Sądej-Sobolewska, Kinga. 2011b. "On the importation of *river* into English". In: Jacek Fisiak — Magdalena Bator (eds.) *Foreign Influences on Medieval English.* Frankfurt am Main: Peter Lang Verlag. 315–326.

Sądej-Sobolewska, Kinga. 2012. "*Tide* and *time* in Middle English dialects". In: Joanna Esquibel — Anna Wojtyś (eds.) *Explorations in the English Language: Middle Ages and Beyond. Festschrift for Professor Jerzy Wełna on the Occasion of his 70th Birthday.* Frankfurt am Main: Peter Lang. 229–238.

Sądej-Sobolewska, Kinga — Marta Sylwanowicz. 2011. "Cleanliness is next to godliness: the lexis of personal hygiene and beauty in Old and Middle English". *Kwartalnik Neofilologiczny* 58.1: 69–80.

Schäfer, Jürgen. 1989. *Early Modern English Lexicography, Vol. 2. Additions and Corrections to the OED.* Oxford: Clarendon Press.

Schöffler, Herbert (ed.). 1919. *Beiträge zur mittelenglischen Medizinlitteratur, III* (*Anglistische Abteilung*, Heft 1). Leipzig: Niemeyer.

Scott-Macnab, David. 2013. "The names of all manner of hounds: A unique inventory in a fifteenth-century manuscript". *Viator* 44: 339–368.

Scott-Macnab, David. 2014. "Unrecorded Middle English lexical items in the fifteenth-century treatise, Medicines for Horses: A Preliminary Study". *Notes and Queries* 61: 344–349.

Scott-Macnab, David (ed.). 2003. *A Sporting Lexicon of the Fifteenth Century: The 'J.B. Treatise'* (*Medium Ævum Monographs* 23). Oxford: The Society for the Study of Medieval Languages and Literature.

Serjeantson, Mary S. 1935. *A History of Foreign Words in English*. London: Routledge & Kegan Paul Ltd.

Serjeantson, Mary S. 1938. "The vocabulary of cookery in the fifteenth century". *Essays & Studies of the English Association* 23: 25–37.

Singer, Dorothea W. 1919. "Survey of the medical manuscripts in the British Isles dating from before the sixteenth century". *Proceedings of the Royal Society of Medicine* 12 (Section of the History of Medicine): 96–107.

Siraisi, Nancy G. 1990. *Medieval and Early Renaissance Medicine: An Introduction to Knowledge and Practice*. Chicago/London: University of Chicago Press.

Stannard, Jerry. 1982. "Rezeptliteratur as Fachliteratur". In: William Eamon (ed.) *Studies on Medieval Fachliteratur.* Brussels: Omirel. 59–73.

Strang, Barbara. 1970. *A History of English*. London: Methuen.

Svensson, Ann-Marie. 1997. *Middle English Words for 'town': A Study of Changes in a Semantic Field.* Göteborg: Acta Universitatis Gothoburgensis.

Svensson, Ann-Marie — Jürgen Hering. 2010. "From Germanic 'fence' to 'urban settlement': On the semantic development of English *town*". In: Robert A. Cloutier — Anne Marie Hamilton-Brehn — William A. Kretzschmar, Jr. (eds.) *Studies in the History of the English Language V: Variation and Change in English Grammar and Lexicon: Contemporary Approaches*. Berlin/New York: Walter de Gruyter. 187–201.

Sylvester, Louise M. 2000. "Naming and avoiding naming objects of terror: a case study". In: Irma Taavitsainen — Terttu Nevalainen — Päivi Pahta — Matti Rissanen (eds.) *Placing Middle English in Context*. Berlin/New York: Mouton de Gruyter. 277–292.

Sylvester, Louise M. 2012. "Mining for gold: investigating a semantic classification in the lexis of cloth and clothing". In: Robin Netherton — Gale R. Owen-Crocker (eds.) *Medieval Clothing and Textiles.* Vol. 8. Woodbridge: Boydell Press. 66–82.

Sylvester, Louise — Jane A. Roberts. 2000. *Middle English Word Studies: A Word and Author Index.* Cambridge: D.S. Brewer.

Sylvester, Louise M. — Mark Chambers — Gale R. Owen-Crocker (eds.). 2014. *Medieval Dress and Textiles in Britain: A Multilingual Sourcebook.* Woodbridge: Boydell Press.

Sylwanowicz, Marta. 2003. "Leech, doctor, physician: on the loss of prototypical meanings". *Anglica* 13: 151–164.

Sylwanowicz, Marta. 2006. "Medieval madness: The Anglo-Saxon terminology of mental diseases". *Anglica* 15: 117–129.

Sylwanowicz, Marta. 2007. "Madfolkes and Lunaticke persons…: the synonyms of madness in Old and Middle English texts". *Anglica* 16: 173–183.

Sylwanowicz, Marta. 2009. "It is to be heled with medicines…: Names of medicines in Late Middle English medical texts". *Kwartalnik Neofilologiczny* 56.3: 349–362.

Sylwanowicz, Marta. 2011. "*And this is a wonderful instrument…*: names of surgical instruments in Late Middle English texts". *Anglica* 16: 173–183.

Sylwanowicz, Marta. 2012. "Clene inwit or fule saule? A study of evaluative developments in the domain of CLEANLINESS". In: Joanna Esquibel — Anna Wojtyś (eds.) *Explorations in the English Language: Middle Ages and Beyond. Festschrift for Professor Jerzy Wełna on the Occasion of his 70th Birthday.* Frankfurt am Main: Peter Lang. 339–351.

Sylwanowicz, Marta. 2014a. *Old and Middle English Sickness-nouns in Historical Perspective. A Lexico-Semantic Analysis.* (*Warsaw Studies in English Historical Linguistics* 1). San Diego: Æ Academic Publishing.

Sylwanowicz, Marta. 2014b. "*Here begynnyth and tellyth howe a manschal make hys salves, oynementes and vnguentys.* Towards standard medical terminology in Middle English". *Kwartalnik Neofilologiczny* 61.3: 559–568.

Sylwanowicz, Marta. 2015. "Ways of introducing specialised terminology in Middle English medical recipes". *Kwartalnik Neofilologiczny* 62.4: 585–594.

Sylwanowicz, Marta. 2016. "*And þan it wole be a good oynement restoratif...* Pre- and postnominal adjectives in Middle English medical recipes". *Anglica* 25.2: 57–71.

Sylwanowicz, Marta. 2017a. "Medieval medical writings and their readers: communication of knowledge in Middle English medical recipes". *Linguistica Silesiana* 38: 112–124.

Sylwanowicz, Marta. 2017b. "Noun phrase modification in Early Modern English recipes". *Anglica* 26.2: 37–49.

Taavitsainen, Irma. 1997. "Genre conventions: Personal affect in fiction and non-fiction". In: Matti Rissanen et al. (eds.) *English in Transition. Corpus-based Studies in Linguistic Variation and Genre Styles.* Berlin/New York: Mouton de Gruyter.

Taavitsainen, Irma. 2001. "Middle English recipes. Genre characteristics, text type features and underlying traditions of writing". *Journal of Historical Pragmatics* 2.1: 85–113.

Taavitsainen, Irma — Päivi Pahta (eds.). 2004. *Medical and Scientific Writing in Late Medieval English.* Cambridge: Cambridge University Press.

Tajima, Matsuji. 1988. *Old and Middle English Language Studies: A Classified Bibliography, 1923–1985.* Amsterdam/Philadelphia: John Benjamins Publishing.

Talbot, Charles H. 1967. *Medicine in Medieval England.* London: Oldbourn.

Tani, Akinobu. 2010. Word Pairs in Late Middle English Prose. Unpublished PhD thesis. University of Glasgow.

Tavormina, Teresa M. 2009. "Practice, theory and authority in a Middle English medical text: "Barton's Urines Which He Treated at Tilney"". *Journal of Nephrology* 22: 33–41.

Taylor, Kevin M.G. — Geoffrey Harding. 2005. *Pharmacy Practice.* New York: Taylor & Francis.

Taylor, Robert B. 2008. *White Coat Tales: Medicine's Heroes, Heritage, and Misadventures.* New York: Springer.

Thompson, C.J.S. 1929. *The Mystery and Art of the Apothecary.* Philadelphia: J. B. Lippincott Company.

Thuresson, Bertil. 1950. *Middle English Occupational Terms.* (*Lund Studies in English* 19.) Lund: Gleerup.

Tiersma, Peter M. 1999. *Legal Language.* Chicago: University of Chicago Press.

Voigts, Linda. 1979. "Anglo-Saxon plant remedies and the Anglo-Saxons". *Isis* 70: 250–268.

Voigts, Linda. 1982. "Editing Middle English medical texts: Needs and issues". In: Levere, Trevor (ed.) *Editing Texts in the History of Science and Medicine: Papers given at the Seventeenth Annual Conference on Editorial Problems*, University of Toronto, 6–7 November 1981. New York/London: Garland. 39–68.

Voigts, Linda — Michael R. McVaugh. 1984. "A Latin technical phlebotomy and its Middle English translation". *Transactions of American Philosophical Society* 74.2: 1–69.

Wallner, Björn. 1964a. "Sketch of Guy de Chauliac". In: Wallner, Björn (ed.) *The Middle English Translation of Guy de Chauliac's "Anatomy", with Guy's Essay on the History of Medicine.* (*Lunds Universitets Årsskrift, N. F. 1*, Vol. 56, No. 5.). Lund: Gleerup. xiii–xviii.

Wallner, Björn. 1964b. "Lexical matter in the Middle English translation of Guy de Chauliac". *English Studies* 45: 151–156.

Wallner, Björn. 1969. "A note on some Middle English medical terms". *English Studies* 50: 499–503.

Wallner, Björn. 1987. "On the.i. periphrasis in the N.Y. Chauliac". *Neuphilologische Mitteilungen* 88: 286–294.

Wallner, Björn. 1992. "Plant names in the Middle English Guy de Chauliac". *Studia Neophilologica* 64: 35–44.

Wallis, Faith. 2010. *Medieval Medicine. A Reader.* Toronto: University of Toronto Press.

Wangensteen, Owen H. — Sarah D. Wangensteen. 1979. *Rise of Surgery. From Empiric Craft to Scientific Discipline.* Minneapolis: University of Minnesota Press.

Wear, Andrew. 2000. *Knowledge and Practice in English Medicine, 1550–1680.* Cambridge: Cambridge University Press.

Webster, LiAnne C. 2014. *Pharmacy Practice Today for the Pharmacy Technician.* St. Louis: Elsevier Health Sciences.

Wełna, Jerzy. 1996. *English Historical Morphology.* Warszawa: Wydawnictwa Uniwersytetu Warszawskiego.

Wełna, Jerzy. 2005. "Nim or take? A competition between two high frequency verbs in Middle English". *Studia Anglica Posnaniensia* 41: 53–69.

Wełna, Jerzy. 2009. "The rivalry of *evil, bad* and *ill* in medieval drama". *Kwartalnik Neofilologiczny* 56.3: 329–338.

Yngve, Victor H. 1975. "Depth and historical change of the English genitive". *Journal of English Linguistics* 9: 47–57.

Zebroski, Bob. 2016. *A Brief History of Pharmacy. Humanity's Search for Wellness.* New York/London: Routledge Taylor & Francis Group.

Zimmermann, E. L. 1937. "An early English manuscript on syphilis: A fragmentary translation from the second edition of Gaspar Torrella's Tractatus cum consiliis contra pudendagram seu morbum gallicum". *Bulletin of the History of Medicine* 5: 461–471.

Zimmerman, Leo M. — Ilza Veith. 1993. *Great Ideas in the History of Surgery.* San Francisco: Norman Publishing.

Appendix A

The following list includes terms discussed in chapters three and four. The first group includes references to 'any substance or preparation used in the treatment of disease' (OED, *medicine* n.[1]) in general, i.e. lexemes that could be used as potential primary terms for the lexical category 'medical preparations'. In the second category, the nouns are divided according to dosage form they represent. As stated in chapter one, the spelling of the forms is in accordance with the strategy adopted by the editor of the *Dictionary of Medical Vocabulary in English, 1375–1550,* i.e. (i) only the commonest spelling variant is given (for all the variants DMVE, MED, OED, MEMT and text editions can be consulted), (ii) if the medieval form is close to the corresponding PDE term then the modern form is given (e.g. ME *plaester, plaestre, plaister, playster*, etc. are given as *plaster*), (iii) terms adopted from Latin are given in their original form (e.g. *oleum*, *trochiscus*, *unguentum*).

I. General terms denoting medical preparations:
   antidote, boot, confection, help, helping, medicine, receipt, remedy, spice.

II. Terms denoting dosage forms:
   - **(i) semisolid preparations**: *anointment, balm, electuary, electuarium, emplaster, emplastrum, entrete, grease, lectuary, liniment, ointment, ointure, paste, plaster, potage$_1$, pultes, salve, treat, uncture, unement, unguent, unguentum;*
   - **(ii) solid preparations**: *ball, pellet, pessary, pill, pilule, powder, pulvis, pulver, suppository, trochisk;*
   - **(iii) liquid preparations**: *decoccioun, drink, liquor, oil, potion, potage$_2$, syrup, water.*

Appendix B

Terms denoting specifics

The list includes all references to medical preparations that denote specifics, discussed in chapter five. Within each category (simplex terms and derivatives, compounds and phrases) the material is divided into groups (as established in chapter five), i.e. names indicating the ingredients, origin of the preparation, part of the body or medical condition, therapeutic methods (only simplex terms and derivatives), properties of the preparation, and miscellaneous forms. Because there are often more references to the same medical mixture, such examples are listed together, e.g., *diaborage* (*diaboraginatum, diaboraginum, diaborago*). In the group of compounds and phrases, the combinations with *of*-phrase (if there are any) will come first as their forms are closer to present-day equivalents, while their equivalent forms will be put in alphabetical order in brackets, e.g., *oil of violet(s)* (*oil de violet, oil violet, oleum violace*). For the exact meaning of each name one should consult available dictionaries (DMVE, MED, OED).

Simplex terms and derivatives

I. **Names indicating the main ingredients**:

(i) **ingredients of plant origin**: *damaceo, diaborage* (*diaboraginatum, diaboraginum, diaborago*), *diabuglosse, diacalamentum, diacamedreos, diacapparis, diacarthamus, diacassiafistula, diaceraseos, diaciminum* (*diacinimum*), *diacison, diacitoniten* (*diacitoniton*), *diacodion, diacoston* (*diacostum*), *diacroca, diaculon* (*diaculum, diaquilon*), *diacuminum, diadactilatum, diadragagant* (*diadragagantum, diadragantum, diagragantum*), *diaflosmus, diagalanga* (*diagalange*), *diagrydie* (*diagrydium*), *diahyssopus, diairis, dialacca* (*dialacce*), *dialibanum* (*diaoliban, diaolibanum*), *dialthe* (*dialthea*), *diamaratrum, diamente, diamirra, diamoron, dianisum, dianthos, dianucum, diapalma, diapapaver, diapenidion, diapigamum, diapiperos* (*diapiperion*), *diaprassion* (*diaprassium*), *diapruna* (*diaprunis*), *diapyrethron* (*diapyrethrum*), *diareubarbare* (*diareubarbarum, diarhubarb*), *diarodon, diasatyrion, diasene, diaspermaticon* (*diaspermaton*), *diaspoliticum, diasquilla, diasymphytum, diatrionpiperon, diaturbith, diazinziber* (*diazinziberis, diazinziberos, diazinziberum*), *glaukin, miclete, opiata* (*opiate, opium*), *pigra, piment, populeon, ptisan* (*tisan*), *rose, sinapism, triasandal* (*triasandri*), *ypoquistid* (*ypoquistidos*).

(ii) **ingredients of animal origin**: *anatison*, *cantharide*, *castoreolon* (*castoreon*), *ceroneum*, *cerote* (*cerotum*), *ciroin*, *diacastorea* (*diacastoreum*), *diamargariton*, *diamber* (*diambra*), *diarundines*, *mel*.

(iii) **ingredients of mineral origin**: *alcofol*, *alfilude*, *aurea*, *diapompholygos*, *emplome*, *nutritum*.

II. **Names indicating the origin of the medicament**:

(i) **medical authorities**: *andromachi*, *marciaton*, *mithridatum*, *philonium*.

(ii) **historical figures**: *adrianum*, *agrippa*, *esdra*, *iustinum*.

(iii) **religious/divine authorities**: *apostolicon*, *theodoricon*.

(iv) **place of origin**: *antioche*, *nerbon*.

III. **Names indicating a body part or medical condition**: *cordial*, *nasale*, *nerval*, *stomaticon*, *sanguiboetos*, *sanguinolent*.

IV. **Names indicating therapeutic methods**: *balneum*, *chewing*, *clyster*, *encatisma*, *enema*, *gargarisma*, *frotting*, *fumigation*, *injection*, *mastication*, *suffumigation*, *stuphe*.

V. **Names indicating the properties of medicaments**

(i) **closing medicines**:

- (a) **astringent medicines**: *aggregative*, *closer*, *conglutinativum*, *conglutinative*, *consouder*, *indurative*, *souder*.
- (b) **cicatrizant medicines**: *cicatrizative*, *consolidative*, *generatif*, *incarnative*, *regenerative*, *sigillative*, *solidative*.

(ii) **constricting medicines**: *constrainative*, *constrictive*, *constrictory*, *restrictive*, *stypter*, *styptic*, *styptica*, *strictory*, *thinner*.

(iii) **opening medicines**: *aperitiva*, *aperitive*, *diaphoretic*, *dilative*, *leptomer*, *liptomer*.

(iv) **cleansing medicines**: *ablution*, *abstersive*, *cleanser*, *lavament*, *lavatory*, *mundyficative*, *mundifier*, *saramitum*, *washer*, *washing*.

(v) **purging medicines**: *attractive*, *catharticum*, *cholagogue*, *deoppilative*, *digestion*, *digestive*, *diuretic*, *diuretica*, *drawer*, *eductive*, *evacuative*, *evaporative*, *expressure*, *expulsive*, *extractive*, *fleumagogue* (*fleumagogon*, *fleumagogum*), *fnesing*, *(h)iera*, *laxative*, *melagogue*, *mordificative*, *pharmacy*, *purgacia*, *purgation*, *purgative*, *sternutory*, *sudatorium*, *tractative*, *trifera*, *urinative*, *vaporative*, *vomit*.

(vi) **repercussive medicines**: *apocrustica*, *blisterer*, *consumentia*, *consumptive*, *impulsive*, *(re)percussif*, *rebounder*, *repercussion*, *repercussive*, *repercussivum*, *repulsive*, *restrainer*, *stupefactive*, *treacle*, *waster*.

(vii) **corrosive medicines**: *aldaron, breaker, capitel, capitellum, caustic, cauterisative, corrosive, corsie, fretter, martencium, mordicative, mortificative, putrefactive, ruptory, ulcerative.*

(viii) **dissolving medicines**: *colliquatif, dissolutifice, dissolutive, dissolventia, incisiva, inscisive, resolutive.*

(ix) **reducing medicines**: *attenuancia, extenuative, rarestiva, rarifactive, subtiliative.*

(x) **drying medicines**: *dessicantia, dessicative, dryer, exsiccative, siccative.*

(xi) **moistening medicines**: *humectantia, moister.*

(xii) **suppurative medicines**: *maturativa, maturative, riper, suppurative.*

(xiii) **palliative medicines**: *abater, anodyna, assuager, comfortative, comforter, dwale, mitigative, narcotic, narcoticum, relaxative, requies, sedative, soporative, swager.*

(xiv) **mollifying medicines**: *bath, epithema, epithemation, foment, fomentation, lenificative, lenitive, lesser, molliative, mollificative, mollifier, mollitive, remollitive, softer, softener, suppler.*

(xv) **heating medicines**: *calefaciencia, calefaction, calefactory, calefactive, chafer.*

(xvi) **cooling medicines**: *enfreider, extinguentia, frigidative, infreider, infrigidatif, keeler, refrigerative.*

(xvii) **preventive medicines**: *conditum, conservative, defender, defending, defensive, preservative, refrainer, refrenative.*

(xviii) **restorative medicines**: *acutives, fastener, illuminative, restaurative, restorative, resumptive, sanative.*

(xix) **alterative medicines**: *alterative, alterer.*

(xx) **topical medicines**: *local.*

(xxi) **colour of the medicine**: *blanca, rubea.*

(xxii) **special attributes of a medicine**: *benedicta.*

(xxiii) **other properties**: *knittere, leader, preparative, provoker, straining.*

VI. Miscellaneous

acaristum, alcalcolon, antamaron, aragon, athanasia, basilicon, burud, cataplasm, claret, climax, colature, collyrie (*collyrium*)*, colman, combrota,* (*dia*)*catholicon, deute, diacomeron, diatesseroun, dradge, euperisten, gommery, grace, gruel, julep, litontripon, lycium, magdaleon, mead, opopira, ordeatum, philantropos, qvadrineroun, sape, sief, sorifilon, stephannia, tetrapharmaca, tincture, triapharmacum, tryufiloun, valence, verlilium.*

Compounds and phrases

I. Names indicating the main ingredients

(i) ingredients of plant origin: *acetum squilliticum, aqua gariofilata, aqua salgie, ball of aloes (pilule of aloe, pilule of aloes), ball of fumitory (pilule of fumtory, pilule de fumo terre), ball of wild celandine, basilicon minus (less basilicon), bean water, ciroin of roses, confectio anacardina, conserve citoniorum, conserve of comfrey, conserve of roses (conserve rosarum), electuarium de succo rosarum, electuarium psilliticum, electuary de boccis lauri, electuary of roses, emplaster of acorus (plaster of acorus, emplastrum de acoro), emplaster of betony (plaster of betony, emplastrum capitale of betony, emplastrum betonice), emplaster of camomile, emplaster diaflosmus, emplaster of diaquilon (emplaster diaquilon, emplastrum diaquilon), emplaster of the two granates (emplaster of two pomegranates, plaster of two granates), emplaster of hocks, emplaster of hollyhock, emplaster of ireos, emplaster of leeks, emplastrum of leek, emplaster of mallows, emplaster of mustard seed (plaster of mustard seed), emplaster of plantain (emplaster of arnoglossa, emplastrum de arnoglossa, plaster of plantain), emplaster of rosis, emplaster of spica (emplaster de spica, plaster of spikenard), emplaster of ache (emplastrum de apio), emplastrum diapalma, emplaster diatarascos, emplastrum diaceraseos, emplastrum ebulinum, emplastrum euphorbium, fomentacion of rosis, ireate diaquilon, madder water (aqua rubia), maturatif of diaquilon, mel anacardi, mel roset, mel rosaum, more basilicon, oil anacardine (oleum anacardinum), oil de ben (oleum de ben), oil of alkanet (oleum alkanne), oil of almonds (oil of amigdales, oile amigdalarum), oil of anise (oil of anet, oil de dill, oleum aneti, oleum anetinum, oleum humanicum), oil of aristologia, oil of ashes (oleum fraxinum), oil of bitter almonds (oil of sour almonds), oil of broom (oleum geneste, oleum genestinum), oil of camomile (oleum camomille, oleum de camomille), oil of carthamus, oil of chesboll, oil of chrysomels, oil of citonies (oil of citoniorum), oil of cost (oil costine, oleum costinum), oil of cresses, oil of cucumber, oil of cucurbita, oil of cypre (oleum cyprine), oil of elders (oil sambucine, oleum sambucinum), oil of euphorbine (oleum euphorbii, oleum euphorbium), oil of gentian, oil of gold apple, oil of gourd seed, oil of henbane (oleum jusquiami), oil of hemodactiles, oil of juniper, oil of laurel (oil de laurer, oil de bay, oil laurine, oil lauriol, oleum laureum, oleum laurinum), oil of lentiscus, oil of lily (oleum liliacium, oleum de lilio, oleum de lilio compositum), oil of linseed (oleum line), oil of mandragore (oleum mandrage, oleum of mandragore), oil of mastic (oil de mastic, oleum mastice,* *oleum masticics, oleum de mastice), oil of mercury, oil of myrt (oleum myrtinum), oil of nardine (oil nardine, oleum nardinum), oil of nuts (nut oil), oil of nux indica (oleum nucis indice), oil of omphacine (oleum omphacinum), oil of peritory, oil of pitch, oil of poppy, oil of puliol (oleum pulegium, puliol oil), oil of radish (oil of rapes, rape oil), oil of resin, oil of rose(s) (oil of roset, oil de roses, oil rosarum, oil rose oil rosat, oleum rosaceum, oleum rosarum, oleum roses), oil of rue, oil of savin, oil of senvy (oleum de sinapi), oil of sisamite (oil sisamine, oleum sesaminum, oil of cockle), oil of sorrel, oil of spica (oil de spica, oil of spikenard, oleum de spica), oil of stavesacre, oil of turpentine, oil of violet(s) (oil de violet, oil violet, oleum violace, oleum violaceum, oleum violarum), oil of walnuts, oil of wheat, oil of withy, ointment of diuelyn, ointment of mallows (unguentum dialthea), ointment of myrtles (unguentum de mirtillis), ointment populeon (unguentum populeon), oleum camelinum, oleum caprinum, oleum cathapuciarum, oleum celandine, oleum de kerua, oleum de sumac, oleum feni, oleum ladani, oleum malvarum (oleum malvinum), oleum nasturtinum, oleum nenuphar, oleum rutastinum (oleum de ruta), oleum salicis, oleum Syriacum, oxymel of radish, oxymel squill (oxymel squilliticum, squillitic oxymel), pellet of affodil (trochiscus of affodills, trochisk of affodil), pellet of alderon (pellet of aldagaroun, trochiscus aldaron, trochisk of aldaron), pellet of alkekengi, pellet of epithimi, pellet of hermodactilorum, pellet of karobe (trochisk de carob, trochisk of carob), pellet of oak fern (pellet of polypody, trochisk of polypody), pellet of turbith (trochisk de turbith, trochiscus de turbith, trochisk of turbith), pilule fetide, pilule of agaric (pellet de agarico, pilule agaric, pilule de agarico), pilule of bdelium (pilule de bdellio), pilule of euphorbe, pilule of gilofre, pilule of myrobalan (pilule myrobalanorum), pilule of rhubarb, pilule storatiue, plaster of celydone, plaster of centaury (emplastrum de centaurea), plaster of rue, powder of aloes (powder of pigre, pulvis pigre), powder of athanasia, powder of basilicon, powder of baye, powder of daffodils (pulvis affodilli), powder of dragagant, powder of hermodactyls, powder of kerseed, powder of mastic, powder of myrtle(s) (powder of myrtillorum, pulvis of mirtilis), powder of oke tre, powder of peritory, powder of sandragon, powder of scammony, powder of spikenard, powder of the seed of water mint, powder of turbith, rosata nouella, sief de spica, sief de thure, sief of burud, sief of incense, sief memithe, sief rosat, syrup of borage, syrup of bugloss, syrup of calamint, syrup of cucumbers, syrup of fumitory (syrup of fumus terre, syrup de fumo terre, syrupus de fumo terre), syrup of horehound, syrup of hyssop, syrup of jujubes, syrup of langue-de-boeuf, syrup of liquorice, syrup of marjoram, syrup of mint, syrup of myrt (syrup of myrtinus, syrupus myrtinus), syrup of nenuphar (syrup nenuphar, syrupus nenupharie), syrup of plums, syrup of poppy (syrup of papaver, syrupus papaverinus), syrup of quinces, syrup of rose(s) (syrup rosate, syrupus rosaceus, syrupus rosarum), syrup of sene, syrup of sorrel, syrup of spikenard, syrupus of violet (syrupus violaceus simplex, syrupus violarum), syrup of water lily, syrup of wormwood, syrupus diaquilon, syrupus limonum, syrupus squilliticus, trochisk of berberries, tapsimel, tapsivalencia, treacle de boys, treacle diatessaron (tiriaca diatesseron), treacle of asafetida, trochisk of glaucio (trochisk de memitha), trochisk de lactea (trochiscus de lacte), unguentum basilicon, unguentum de ireos, unguentum de palma, unguentum de resina, unguentum de terbentina, unguentum dampnaleon, unguentum diaculum (unguentum diaquilon), unguentum genest(r)e, unguentum lilium, unguentum sompniferum, valence of wormwood, water avenatum, water of agrimony, water of almonds, water of anagallis (water of chicken-meat), water of arnoglossa (water of plantain, plantain water), water of arsesmart, water of avens, water of barley (aqua hordei, aqua ordei), water of betony, water of borage, water of bran, water of bugle, water of caprifoil, water of cauls, water of celidony, water of centaury, water of chervil, water of cicers (water of chiches), water of calamint (calamint water), water of comfrey, water of coriander, water of cucurbita, water of elder, water of endive, water of euphrasy/euphrage, water of fennel (fennel water), water of figs, water of fumitory, water of galls, water of gourds, water of herb bennet, water of herb Robert, water of honeysuckle, water of horehound, water of hyssop, water of ivy, water of langue de boeuf, water of leeks, water of lilies, water of limonum, water of liquorice, water of lye, water of mallow(s), water of marjoram, water of melilot, water of mint(s), water of morel (morel water), water of mouse-ear, water of myrt (aqua mirti), water of nenuphar(s), water of olive(s), water of peony, water of plums, water of poppy, water of radish (water of raphanus), water of ramson(s), water of red fennel, water of red rose (water of rose(s), water of roset, water roset, aqua rosacea, aqua rosarum), water of rue, water of sage, water of sambuci, water of scabious (scabious water), water of scariola, water of seeds, water of shepherd's yard, water of singrene, water of sorrel, water of sperm, water of stanmarch, water of tamarinds, water of tormentil, water of vervain, water of violet(s), water of virga pastoris, water of water lilies, water of water mint, water of white henbane, water of woodbind, water of wormwood, water of worts.*

(ii) **ingredients of animal origin**: *alipta muscata, aqua muscata, confectio alipe muscate, dianthos muscate, confectio gallye muscate, emplaster of a ram's skin, emplaster of ants (emplaster of pismires, emplastrum de formicis), emplaster of the wether's skin, emplastrum ceroneum, oil of castor (oil castorinum), oil of chaunteroil, oil of chicks, oil of dogfish, oil of musceline (oil musceline, oleum muscatelinum, oleum muscelinum), oil of neat's feet, oil of scorpions (oleum scorpionum), oil of serpents, oil of snails, oil of worms, oleum lubrecum, ointment of backs, ointment of fox (unguentum de vulpe), ointment of the gander, pellet of spodium, plaster of sheep's skin, plaster of worms, pilule of castor, pilule of diacastorie (pilule diacastor, pilule diacastoree), potio muscata, powder of castor, powder of clowes, unguentum de ansere, unguentum de vermibus, unguentum muscatum, water of honey (aqua mellis).*

(iii) **ingredients of mineral origin**: *aqua cineris, aqua salmacina, collyrie of lede (collyrium de plumbo), emplaster of armoniaco, emplaster of minerales, emplaster of tartare, litharge nourished (litharge nutrite, lithargyrum nutritum), metalline oinement, mineral oinement, oil of lede (oleum plumby), oil of quick brimstone (oil of sulphur, oleum sulphuris), oil of tar (oil of tartar, oleum tartar, oleum tartari, oleum tartarinum), ointment of bole (oinement of bole armoniac, unguentum de bolo), ointment of litharge, ointment of tutty (unguentum de tuttio), pellet of quicklime (trochisk of lime), pitchy plaster, plaster of plumb (emplaster plumbi, emplastrum plumbi), plaster of ceruse, powder of alumne, powder of arsenek, powder of bole armonac, powder of coral, sal sacerdolate, salt water, sief of hematites, sief of lead (sief de plumbo), sief of vitriol, sief rusceym, trochisk of diabardich, unguentum de calce/calx, unguentum nutritum, water of alum (alum water, alumed water, alumy water, aqua aluminosa), water of argol, water of brimstone, water of copperas, water of flint, water of iron, water of minerals (mineral water), water of salmacina, water of salt, water of sugar (sugar water), water of sulphur (sulphured water, sulphury water, soufry water), water of tartar (water of tartarum), white plaster of ceruse.*

(iv) **other**: *emplastrum oxycroceum, hiera pigra, mellicrate, oil of ey yolks (oil of eyren, oil of eggs), oil of man's dirt, oinement of line (unguentum de lino/line), oxycratum, oxycroceum, oxygranatorum, oxysaccharum, rodozacar, rodoraca, syrup of vinegar (syrupus acetosus, sour syrup), syrup of oxysacchare, syrup of oxymel, syrupus julep, syrupus penidie, water of ashes (aqua saponis, water of soap), water of cheese, water of eyren, water of man's blood, water of the lung.*

II. Names indicating the origin of the medicament

(i) medical authorities: *Alexander's oinement (oinement of Alexander), aromaticon of Hebemesue, auree Alexandrina, Avicenna's diaquilon, Avicenna's powder, black powder of Arnald, cerote of Galen, ciminata alexandrina, diaquilon Rhazes, electuarium Cophonis, electuarium frigidum Cophonis, electuarium laxativum frigidum Cophonis, emplaster capital of Master Anselm of Genoa (chief plaster of Master Anselm of Genoa), emplastrum croceum of Master Petrus de Bonanto, emplastrum fuscum Brademore, Galen's ciroin, Galen's gladding medicine, Galen's green oinement (unguentum viride Galeni), Galen's powder (pulvis Galeni), Galen's wonderful medicine, green ointment of Lanfrank, green plaster of Master Pers de Bonaunt, Master Peter's water of Spain (water of Master Peter), medicine of Haly the Abbot, ieraruffini, leticia Galeni, musa enea, oil marciaton, ointment of Master William Someris, oinement of the Four Masters, pellet of Andronium (trochisk Andronii, trochisk of Andronii), pilule cochie Rhazes (cochie Rasie), pilule Benvenuci, pilule Gallice, powder of Benvenute (Benvenute's powder), powder of Haram, powder of Master Arnald (Master Arnald's powder), powder of Master Dine (Master Dine's powder), powder Walter (pulvis Walteri/Walter), Rhazes' powder (pulvis Rhazes), Rhazes' white plaster, syrup of Platearie, Theodoric's liniment (liniment of Theodoric), tiriaca Galeni, unguent of Master Dine, unguentum album Rhazes, unguentum Aristotilis, unguentum marciaton (unguentum marciatum), unguentum nigrum Haly, unguentum Rhazes, unguentum Stephani, unguentum viride cirurgicorum, yellow plaster of Master Pers de Bonanto, yerapigra constantini, yerapigra galieni, zinziber Alexandrinum.*

(ii) historical figures: *diarrhodon abbatis, electuarium ducis, katarticum imperiale, King's oinement (unguentum regis Anglie), King William oil, potio Adriani, potio Justini, unguentum agrippa/agrippe, unguentum imperiale, water imperial.*

(iii) religious/divine authorities: *angel bread, apostles' plaster (unguentum apostolorum), apostles' plaster (unguentum apostolorum), donum Dei, emplaster apostolicon (emplaster apostolorum, emplastrum apostolicon), emplastrum Gratia Dei (grace of God, Gratia Dei, Gratia Dei maior, Gratia Dei media, more gratia Dei), iera Hermetis, oinement of Mary Magdalene, pilgrim's salve, potio Esdre, potio Sancti Pauli (pocio santi pauly, potio simplicis paulini), theodoricon anacardi (theodoricum anacardinum), theodoricon empericon (theodoricon enperiston), unguentum Nicodemi, unguentum veneris, virtue given of God (virtus a Deo datum).*

(iv) **place of origin**: *bewe of Antioche* (*drink of Antioche, potus Antioche*), *diolibanum Salernitanum, emplaster of Nerbon, emplaster of Montpellier* (*plaster of Montpellier*), *French water* (*aqua gallicana*), *igia Greca, Nabateans' powder* (*pulvis Nabatinus*), *oil of Exeter, ointment of Macedon, pellet of Antioche, pilule of Araby* (*pilule Arabie*), *pilule Iherosolimitane, plaster of Paris, powder of Greek* (*powder Greek, pulver Greke, pulvis Grecus*), *pulvis Assyricus, red plaster of Greek* (*emplastrum rubeum Grecum*), *syrup of Antioche, trifera saracenica, unguentum Arabicum, unguentum Egiptiacum, unguentum judeorum, unguentum Saracenicum.*

(v) **other**: *diarrhodon Julii*, fellow's water, *my father's electuary* (*electuarium patris, electuarium patris mei*), *unguentum viride Almasoris.*

III. **Names indicating body parts or medical condition**: *acute medicine, capital medicine, capital plaster* (*plaster capital*), *capital powder* (*chief powder, pulvis capitalis/capital*), *emplaster nerval* (*emplastrum nerval*), *medicyns þat ben particuler, pilule artetice, potio vulneratorum, powder of stomaticon comfortativum, pulvis stomaticus comfortativus, unguentum nervale, wounded men's drink.*

IV. **Names indicating the properties of medicaments**

(i) **closing medicines**:

(a) **astringent medicines**: *binding medicine, cleaving medicine, consolidative medicine, consolidative oinement* (*consouding oinement*), *consolidative emplaster* (*consolidative plaster*), *consouditive drink, fastening medicine, glutinative medicine, knitting medicine, medicine aggregative, medicine conglutinative, plaster soudinge.*

(b) **cicatrizant medicines**: *cicatrizative medicine, cicatrizing medicine, compressive medicine, emplaster incarnative, fleshing medicine, fleshing ointment, fleshing plaster, healing ointment, healing plaster, incarnative medicine, incarnative ointment, medicina cicatrizativa, medicine cicarnative, medicine generative, medicine regenerative, medicine sigillative, plaster incarnative, powder cicatrizing, powder cicazitrative, powder consolidative, powder incarnative, powder regenerative, pulvis consolidativus, regenerative medicine, souding medicine, souding oinement, souding powder, unguentum consolidativum.*

(ii) **constricting medicines**: *bath strictory, constraining medicine, constraining pellet, constraining plaster, constraining powder, constrictive bath, constrictive emplaster, constrictive medicine, constrictive powder, emplaster binding, emplaster restrictive, emplaster strictive, oil of styptic, oppilative medicine, pillule stiptice, plaster constrictive, plaster restrictive, plaster* *strictory, powder restrictive, restraining medicine, restraining powder, stopping medicine, straining medicine, strictive powder, strictive syrup, strictory medicine, styptic emplaster, styptic medicine, styptic oil, styptic plaster, styptic syrup, styptic water, stypticative medicine, superfluity medicine, syrup constrictive, syrupus stypticus, withstanding medicine.*

(iii) **opening medicines**: *medicine aperitive, medicine diaphoretic, medicine liptomer, oil diaphoretic, opening medicine, unstopping powder.*

(iv) **cleansing medicines**: *abstersive medicine, clarificacio oculorum, clarificative medicine, clarifying powder, cleansing medicine, cleansing oinement, clearing medicine, electuarium þat biþ clensynge, medicine mundificative, mundificative emplaster, plaster mundificative, scouring medicine, unguentum mundificativum, washing medicine.*

(v) **purging medicines**: *attractive lectuary, attractivum emplaster, avoiding medicine, brakeling medicine, caput purgies, catahrticum imperiale, diuretic drink, diuretic medicine, diuretic powder, diuretic syrup, drawing medicine, drawing plaster, drawing salve, emplaster attractive, emplastrum attractivum, evapouring medicine, expulsive medicine, fnesing medicine, lavative medicine, lavative powder, laxative medicine, laxative oxymel, medicine attractive, medicine digestative, medicine digestive, medicine evacuative, medicine evaporative, medicine of digestion, medicine purgative, medicine tractative, medicine unbinding, oinement drawing, oinement laxative, oxymel diuretic, oxymel diureticum, oxymel laxativum, purging medicine, quenching medicine, sal catharticum, spewing medicine, suppository mordificative, syrup digestive, syrup þat is laxative, theodoricon expericito laxativa, vapouring medicine, voiding medicine, vomiting medicine, vomitive medicine.*

(vi) **repercussive medicines**: *antidotum ymagogum, blistering medicine, emplaster repercussive, extirpative medicine, medicine abstractive, medicine (þat beþ) consuming, medicine consumptive, medicine rebounding, plaster spending, plaster wasting, repercussive medicine, straining plaster, wasting medicine.*

(vii) **corrosive medicines**: *adustive medicine, aqua ardent, ardent water, ball of aldaron, ball of calidicon, biting medicine, biting suppository, breaking medicine, breaking ointment, burning medicine, burning water, bursting medicine, corrosive medicine, corrosive water, fretting medicine, fretting oinement, gnawing medicine, medicine caustic, medicine cauterative, medicine cauterizant, medicine cauterizative, medicine of cautering, medicine of putrefaction, medicine ruptive, medicine piercing, oil corrosive, ointment* *corrosive, ointment ruptory, pellet calidicon, pellet of aldaron, pellet of calidicon, powder corrosive, pulvis corrosivus/corrosive, rotting medicine, ruptory unement, scarotic medicine, searing medicine, sharp medicine, shaving medicine, slaying medicine, trochiscus calidicon, trochisc(us) of aldaron, trochisk calidicon, ulcerative medicine, unguentum ruptorium, unguentum viride corrosivum, water ardent.*

(viii) **dissolving medicines**: *aqua fortis, defying medicine, dissolutive medicine, emplaster dissolutive, emplaster resolutive, emplastrum resolutivum, loosing medicine, medicine dissolving, medicine divisive, medicine incisive, oil þat is resolutive, oil þat is resolving, ointment resolutive, oxymel divisivum, potio resoluens, resolving medicine, resolutive plaster, solutive medicine, strong water.*

(ix) **reducing medicines**: *subtiliative medicine, subtling medicine, unguentum subtile.*

(x) **drying medicines**: *desiccative medicine, dry bath, drying emplaster, drying medicine, drying oinement, drying plaster, emplaster dessicative, medicine exsiccative, medicine siccative, ointment dessicative, siccative water, unguentum desiccativum.*

(xi) **moistening medicines**: *electuary humiditative, electuary moisting, medicine humectative, moist medicine, moisting medicine, moist oil, moist ointment, moist plaster.*

(xii) **suppurative medicines**: *maturative emplaster, maturative medicine, maturative plaster, medicine maturing, medicine riping, medicine suppurative, oil þat is maturative, oil þat is ripe, riping emplaster, riping medicine, riping plaster.*

(xiii) **palliative medicines**: *abating medicine, comfortable drink, comfortable electuary, comfortative bath, comfortative medicine, comforting plaster, cordial syrup, dulling medicine, electuarium þat is comfortative, electuary comfortative, electuary confortativum, emplaster comfortative, emplaster þat is mitigative, emplastrum mitigativum, lissing medicine, lissing oil, medicine þat is comfortable, mitigative medicine, mitigative plaster, narcotic medicine, obdormitive medicine, oil calastic, oil mitigative, ointment asauging, powder comforting, powder of stomaticon comfortativum, powder subtle, sedative medicine, sedative oil, slaking medicine, staunching medicine, stomaticon calidum comfortatum, swaging medicine, swaging plaster, unguentum confortativum.*

(xiv) **mollifying medicines**: *liking medicine, mollificative emplaster, mollificative medicine, mollifying medicine, mollitive medicine, neshing medicine,* *oil þat is mollificative, ointment mollificative, plaster mollificative, remolliative oinement, remollitive oinement, softening bath, softening medicine, softening oil, soft plaster, suppling oil, unguentum mollificativum.*

(xv) **heating medicines**: *chafing medicine, medicine heating.*

(xvi) **cooling medicines**: *colding medicine, cooling medicine, electuarium frigidum, electuary frigidum, infrigidative medicine, keeling medicine, oinement þat is keeling, stomaticon frigidum.*

(xvii) **preventive medicines**: *aqua conservativa, forbidding medicine, medicine defensive, medicine preservative, medicine refrenative, powder conservative, refraining medicine.*

(xviii) **restorative medicines**: *batter sanative, electuarium resumptivum, electuarium þat is restaurative, emplaster restaurative, emplaster restorative, medicine restorative, medicine resumptive, ointment restorative, ointment sanative, restoring medicine, restoring ointment, unguentum resumptivum.*

(xix) **alterative medicines**: *changing medicine, cold changing medicine, drink alterative, medicine alterative, syrup alterative.*

(xx) **qualities (hot, cold, dry, moist) of medicines**: *cold diapapaver, cold diuretic, cold electuary, cold emplaster, cold medicine, cold oil, cold ointment, cold pilule, cold plaster, cold syrup, cold water, distemporate medicine, dry medicine, dry syrup, hot electuary, hot emplaster, hot medicine, hot oil, hot ointment, hot plaster, hot powder, meddled medicine, medicine out of temper, temperate medicine, temperate ointment, temporate medicine, temporate oil, unguentum theraticum, untemporate medicine.*

(xxi) **topical medicines**: *local medicine, medicine to the place, adjutorium locale, adjutorium to the place, adjutory to the place.*

(xxii) **medical and surgical medicines**: *chirurgical medicine, physical medicine.*

(xxiii) **colour of a medicine**: *black emplaster, black entrete, black ointment, black plaster, black powder, citrine ointment, citrine powder, citrine sief, common unguentum album, confection nere, double-coloured medicine, dun grey ointment, dun ointment, emplastrum album, emplastrum nigrum, emplastrum rubeum, emplastrum viride, green entrete, green oil, green ointment, green powder, green sief, ointment fusco, ointment of alabaster* (*unguentum alabastri*), *pilule auree, potio rubea, pulvis citrinus, pulver rubeus* (*pulvis rubeus*), *red ointment, red powder, red salve, red sief, red water, rubea trociscata, sief album, sief citrinum, unguentum album, unguentum aureum, unguentum azurin(um), unguentum citrinum, unguentum fuscum, unguentum nigrum, unguentum rubeum, unguentum viridum, unguentum* *viride herbarum, white collyrie, white emplaster, white oil, white ointment, yellow emplaster, yellow ointment, yellow powder.*

(xxiv) **flavour/aroma of a medicine**: *aqua aromatica, aromatic water, electuarium alarfit, electuarium dulce, emplastrum flavum.*

(xxv) **medicines obtained through the infusion of herbs or distillation**: *aqua vite, distilled water, first water, infused water, second water, stilled water, third water, water of life.*

(xxvi) **special attributes of a medicine**: *benedicta potio, diapenidium magnum, emplastrum laudabile, great diaquilon, great treacle, ointment of gleyr, oil bennet, oleum benedictum, pliris arconticon, powder sine pari, precious ointment, pulvis benedictus/benedicte, pulvis pliris tiriaca maior, pulvis sine pari, treacle maior, tricata magna, trifera magna, unguentum glorie, unguentum preciosum, unguentum speciale, unguentum vade mecum, universal medicine, vade mecum, veni mecum.*

V. **Miscellaneous names**: *aqua composita, aqua salutis, balneum eucratum, compound electuarium, compound medicine, electuarium pluris, ironed water, lac virgineum, oxymel compositum, oxymel compound, oxymel simplex, pilule octomere, pilule optomere, powder creoferoberon, powder of creoferoberon, pulver creoferoberon, salus populi, sanc dragans, simple medicine, simple oil, smith's water, suppository provocative, unguentum tetrapharmacum, water of iron.*

Index of terms

Hereafter are listed the names of medical preparations that are discussed in more detail in the present work. The references are to the sections in which the terms are described.

D

Studies in English Medieval Language and Literature

Edited by Jacek Fisiak

Vol. 1 Dieter Kastovsky / Arthur Mettinger (eds.): Language Contact in the History of English. 2nd, revised edition. 2003.

Vol. 2 Studies in English Historical Linguistics and Philology. A Festschrift for Akio Oizumi. Edited by Jacek Fisiak. 2002.

Vol. 3 Liliana Sikorska: *In a Manner of Morall Playe*: Social Ideologies in English Moralities and Interludes (1350-1517). 2002.

Vol. 4 Peter J. Lucas / Angela M. Lucas (eds.): Middle English from Tongue to Text. Selected Papers from the Third International Conference on Middle English: Language and Text, held at Dublin, Ireland, 1-4 July 1999. 2002.

Vol. 5 Chaucer and the Challenges of Medievalism. Studies in Honor of H. A. Kelly. Edited by Donka Minkova and Theresa Tinkle. 2003.

Vol. 6 Hanna Rutkowska: Graphemics and Morphosyntax in the *Cely Letters* (1472-88). 2003.

Vol. 7 The *Ancrene Wisse*. A Four-Manuscript Parallel Text. Preface and Parts 1-4. Edited by Tadao Kubouchi and Keiko Ikegami with John Scahill, Shoko Ono, Harumi Tanabe, Yoshiko Ota, Ayako Kobayashi and Koichi Nakamura. 2003.

Vol. 8 Joanna Bugaj: Middle Scots Inflectional System in the South-west of Scotland. 2004.

Vol. 9 Rafal Boryslawski: The Old English Riddles and the Riddlic Elements of Old English Poetry. 2004.

Vol. 10 Nikolaus Ritt / Herbert Schendl (eds.): Rethinking Middle English. Linguistic and Literary Approaches. 2005.

Vol. 11 The *Ancrene Wisse*. A Four-Manuscript Parallel Text. Parts 5–8 with Wordlists. Edited by Tadao Kubouchi and Keiko Ikegami with John Scahill, Shoko Ono, Harumi Tanabe, Yoshiko Ota, Ayako Kobayashi, Koichi Nakamura. 2005.

Vol. 12 Text and Language in Medieval English Prose. A Festschrift for Tadao Kubouchi. Edited by Akio Oizumi, Jacek Fisiak and John Scahill. 2005.

Vol. 13 Michiko Ogura (ed.): Textual and Contextual Studies in Medieval English. Towards the Reunion of Linguistics and Philology. 2006.

Vol. 14 Keiko Hamaguchi: Non-European Women in Chaucer. A Postcolonial Study. 2006.

Vol. 15 Ursula Schaefer (ed.): The Beginnings of Standardization. Language and Culture in Fourteenth-Century England. 2006.

Vol. 16 Nikolaus Ritt / Herbert Schendl / Christiane Dalton-Puffer / Dieter Kastovsky (eds): Medieval English and its Heritage. Structure, Meaning and Mechanisms of Change. 2006.

Vol. 17 Matylda Włodarczyk: Pragmatic Aspects of Reported Speech. The Case of Early Modern English Courtroom Discourse. 2007.

Vol. 18 Hans Sauer / Renate Bauer (eds.): *Beowulf* and Beyond. 2007.

Vol. 19 Gabriella Mazzon (ed.): Studies in Middle English Forms and Meanings. 2007.

Vol. 20 Alexander Bergs / Janne Skaffari (eds.): The Language of the Peterborough Chronicle. 2007.

Vol. 21 Liliana Sikorska (ed.). With the assistance of Joanna Maciulewicz: Medievalisms. The Poetics of Literary Re-Reading. 2008.

Vol. 22 Masachiyo Amano / Michiko Ogura / Masayuki Ohkado (eds.): Historical Englishes in Varieties of Texts and Contexts. The Global COE Program, International Conference 2007. 2008.

Vol. 23 Ewa Ciszek: Word Derivation in Early Middle English. 2008.

Vol. 24 Andrzej M. Łęcki: Grammaticalisation Paths of *Have* in English. 2010.

Vol. 25 Osamu Imahayashi / Yoshiyuki Nakao / Michiko Ogura (eds.): Aspects of the History of English Language and Literature. Selected Papers Read at SHELL 2009, Hiroshima. 2010.

Vol. 26 Magdalena Bator: Obsolete Scandinavian Loanwords in English. 2010.

Vol. 27 Anna Cichosz: The Influence of Text Type on Word Order of Old Germanic Languages. A Corpus-Based Contrastive Study of Old English and Old High German. 2010.

Vol. 28 Jacek Fisiak / Magdalena Bator (eds.): Foreign Influences on Medieval English. 2011.

Vol. 29 Władysław Witalisz: The Trojan Mirror. Middle English Narratives of Troy as Books of Princely Advice. 2011.

Vol. 30 Luis Iglesias-Rábade: Semantic Erosion of Middle English Prepositions. 2011.

Vol. 31 Barbara Kowalik: Betwixt *engelaunde* and *englene londe*. Dialogic Poetics in Early English Religious Lyric. 2010.

Vol. 32 The Katherine Group. A Three-Manuscript Parallel Text. Seinte Katerine, Seinte Marherete, Seinte Iuliene, and Hali Meiðhad, with Wordlists. Edited by Shoko Ono and John Scahill with Keiko Ikegami, Tadao Kubouchi, Harumi Tanabe, Koichi Nakamura, Satoko Shimazaki and Koichi Kano. 2011.

Vol. 33 Jacob Thaisen / Hanna Rutkowska (eds.): Scribes, Printers, and the Accidentals of their Texts. 2011.

Vol. 34 Isabel Moskowich: Language Contact and Vocabulary Enrichment. Scandinavian Elements in Middle English. 2012.

Vol. 35 Joanna Esquibel / Anna Wojtyś (eds.): Explorations in the English Language: Middle Ages and Beyond. Festschrift for Professor Jerzy Wełna on the Occasion of his 70th Birthday. 2012.

Vol. 36 Yoshiyuki Nakao: The Structure of Chaucer´s Ambiguity. 2013.

Vol. 37 Begoña Crespo: Change in Life, Change in Language. A Semantic Approach to the History of English. 2013.

Vol. 38 Richard Dance / Laura Wright (eds.): The Use and Development of Middle English. Proceedings of the Sixth International Conference on Middle English, Cambridge 2008. 2012.

Vol. 39 Michiko Ogura: Words and Expressions of Emotion in Medieval English. 2013.

Vol. 40 Anna Czarnowus: Fantasies of the Other´s Body in Middle English Oriental Romance. 2013.

Vol. 41 Hans Sauer / Gaby Waxenberger (eds.): Recording English, Researching English, Transforming English. With the Assistance of Veronika Traidl. 2013.

Vol. 42 Michio Hosaka / Michiko Ogura / Hironori Suzuki / Akinobu Tani (eds.): Phases of the History of English. Selection of Papers Read at SHELL 2012. 2013.

Vol. 43 Vlatko Broz: Aspectual Prefixes in Early English. 2014.

Vol. 44 Michael Bilynsky (ed.): Studies in Middle English. Words, Forms, Senses and Texts. 2014.

Vol. 45 Bożena Duda: The Synonyms of *Fallen Woman* in the History of the English Language. 2014.

Vol. 46 Magdalena Bator: Culinary verbs in Middle English. 2014.

Vol. 47 Juan Camilo Conde-Silvestre / Javier Calle-Martín (eds.): Approaches to Middle English. Variation, Contact and Change. 2015.

Vol. 48 *Sawles Warde* and the Wooing Group. Parallel Texts with Notes and Wordlists. Edited by Harumi Tanabe and John Scahill with Shoko Ono, Keiko Ikegami, Satoko Shimazaki and Koichi Kano. 2015.

Vol. 49 Jacek Fisiak / Magdalena Bator / Marta Sylwanowicz (eds.): Essays and Studies in Middle English. 9th International Conference on Middle English, Philological School of Higher Education in Wrocław, 2015. 2017.

Vol. 50 Ewa Ciszek-Kiliszewska: Middle English Prepositions and Adverbs with the Prefix *be-* in Prose Texts. A Study in Their Semantics, Dialectology and Frequency. 2017.

Vol. 51 Anna Wojtyś: The Non-Surviving Preterite-Present Verbs in English. The Demise of **dugan, munan, *-nugan, *þurfan,* and *unnan*. 2017.

Vol. 52 Harumi Tanabe / Koichi Kano / John Scahill (eds.): Linguistic Variation in the *Ancrene Wisse*, Katherine Group and Wooing Group. Essays Celebrating the Completion of the Parallel Text Edition. 2018.

Vol. 53 Marta Sylwanowicz: Middle English Names of Medical Preparations. Towards a Standard Medical Terminology. 2018.

www.peterlang.com